DOWNLOAD MUSIC & AUDIO
 AbridgeClub.com | Amazon.com | iTunes
DESCARGA MÚSICA y AUDIO
 AbridgeClub.com | Amazon.com | iTunes

We Eat Food That's Fresh!
¡Comemos Comida Fresca!

Written by   La Autora
Angela Russ-Ayon

Illustrated by   La Illustradora
Cathy June

Published and Produced by
Russ InVision

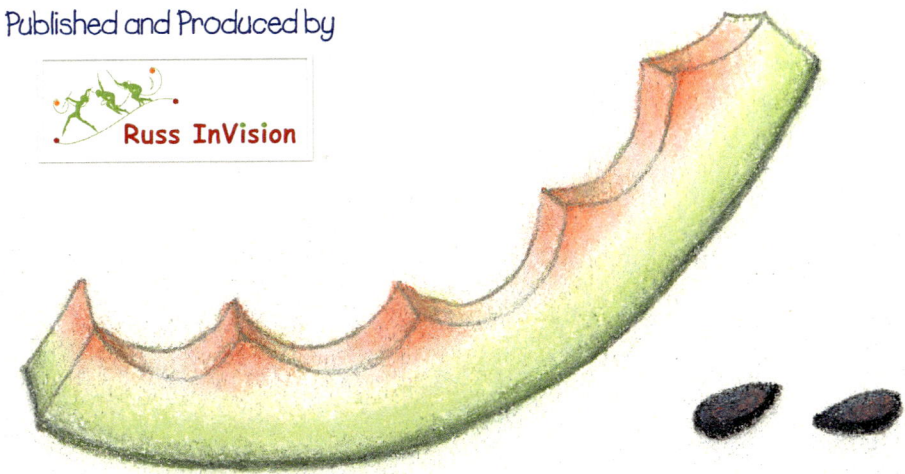

Translation   Traducción
Mercedes Seraphim

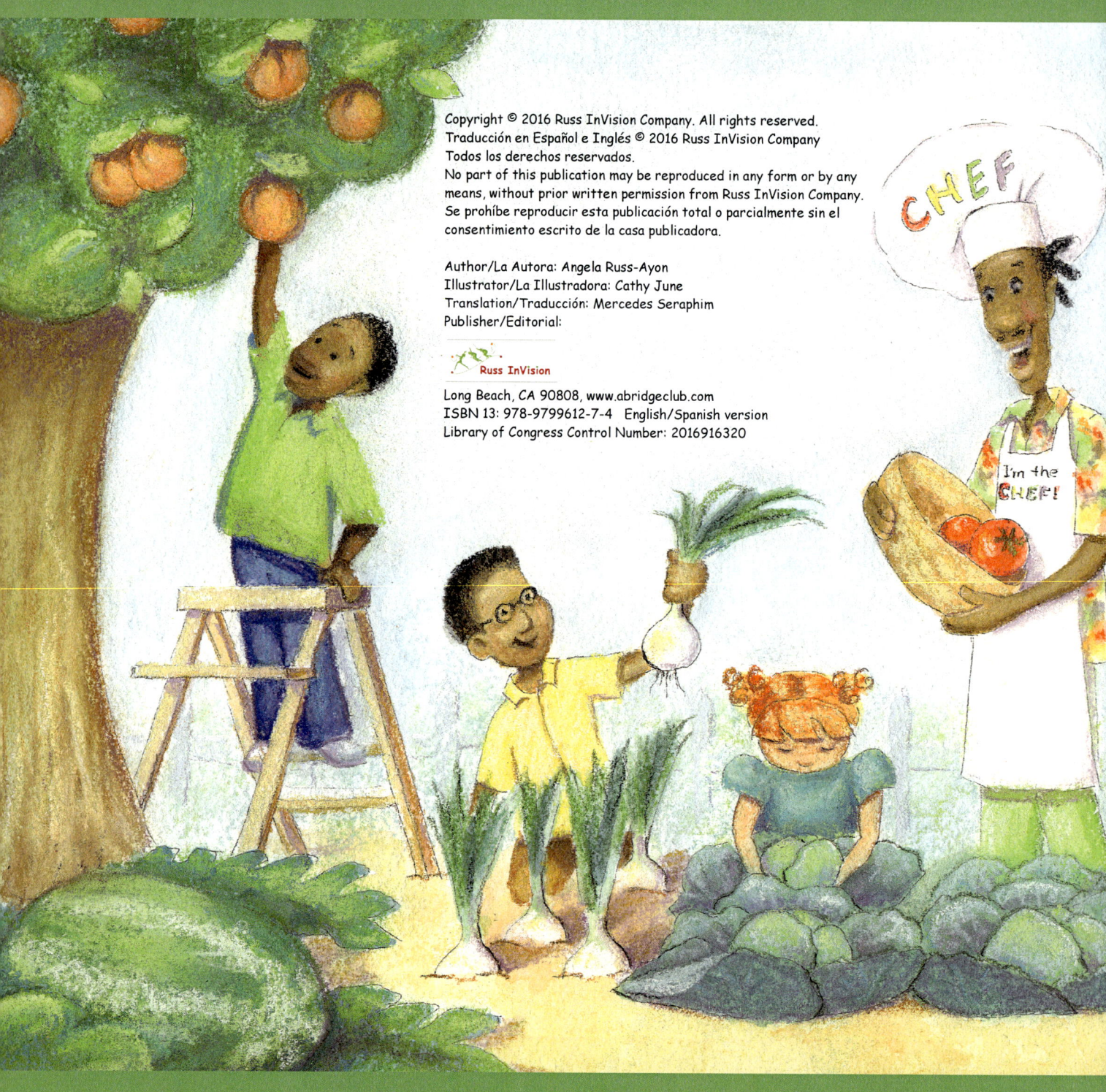

Copyright © 2016 Russ InVision Company. All rights reserved.
Traducción en Español e Inglés © 2016 Russ InVision Company
Todos los derechos reservados.
No part of this publication may be reproduced in any form or by any means, without prior written permission from Russ InVision Company.
Se prohíbe reproducir esta publicación total o parcialmente sin el consentimiento escrito de la casa publicadora.

Author/La Autora: Angela Russ-Ayon
Illustrator/La Illustradora: Cathy June
Translation/Traducción: Mercedes Seraphim
Publisher/Editorial:

Russ InVision

Long Beach, CA 90808, www.abridgeclub.com
ISBN 13: 978-9799612-7-4   English/Spanish version
Library of Congress Control Number: 2016916320

"A simply edible book tha is rich in colorful fruits and vegetables. Inspires all ages to have a taste of something new!"
-Produce For Better Health Foundation, www.MoreMatters.org

Names: Russ-Ayon, Angela, author | June, Cathy, illustrator.
Title: Comemos comida fresca = We eat food that's fresh! / written by Angela Russ-Ayon; illustrated by Cathy June.
Summary: A chef shows children the variety of ways fruits and vegetables can be prepared in order to encourage them to try something new and eat healthy foods.
Description: Long Beach, CA: Russ InVision Company, 2016.
Identifiers: ISBN 978-0-9799612-7-4 | LCCN 2016916320
Subjects: LCSH Nutrition—Juvenile literature. | Diet—Juvenile literature. | Food—Juvenile literature. | Cookery—Juvenile literature. | Fruit—Juvenile literature | Vegetables—Juvenile literature. | Health—Juvenile literature. | BISAC JUVENILE FICTION / Cooking & Food | JUVENILE FICTION / Health & Daily Living / General
Classification: LCC PZ7.R8999 Co 2016 | DDC [E]—dc23

Other titles by this author:

We Eat Food That's Fresh | English
When You Find Colors and Shapes | English
Cuando Encuentres los Colores y las Formas | Spanish and English
Quand Vous Trouvez les Couleurs et les Formes | French and English
We Love the Company, A Book About Table Manners, with Companion CD | English
Fruits and Veggies Making Faces | English
Chalk It up: Outdoor Activities for Early Childhood and Beyond | English

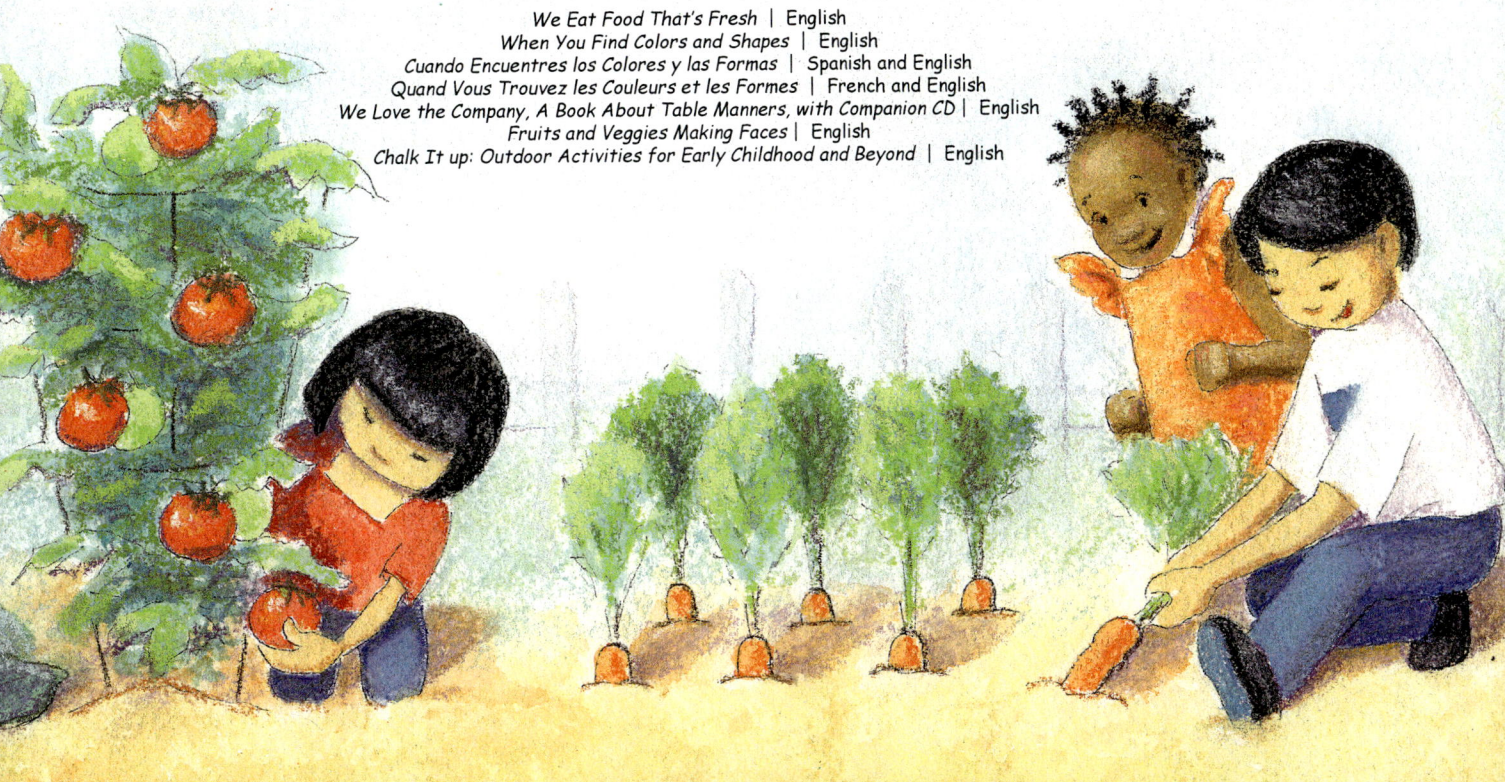

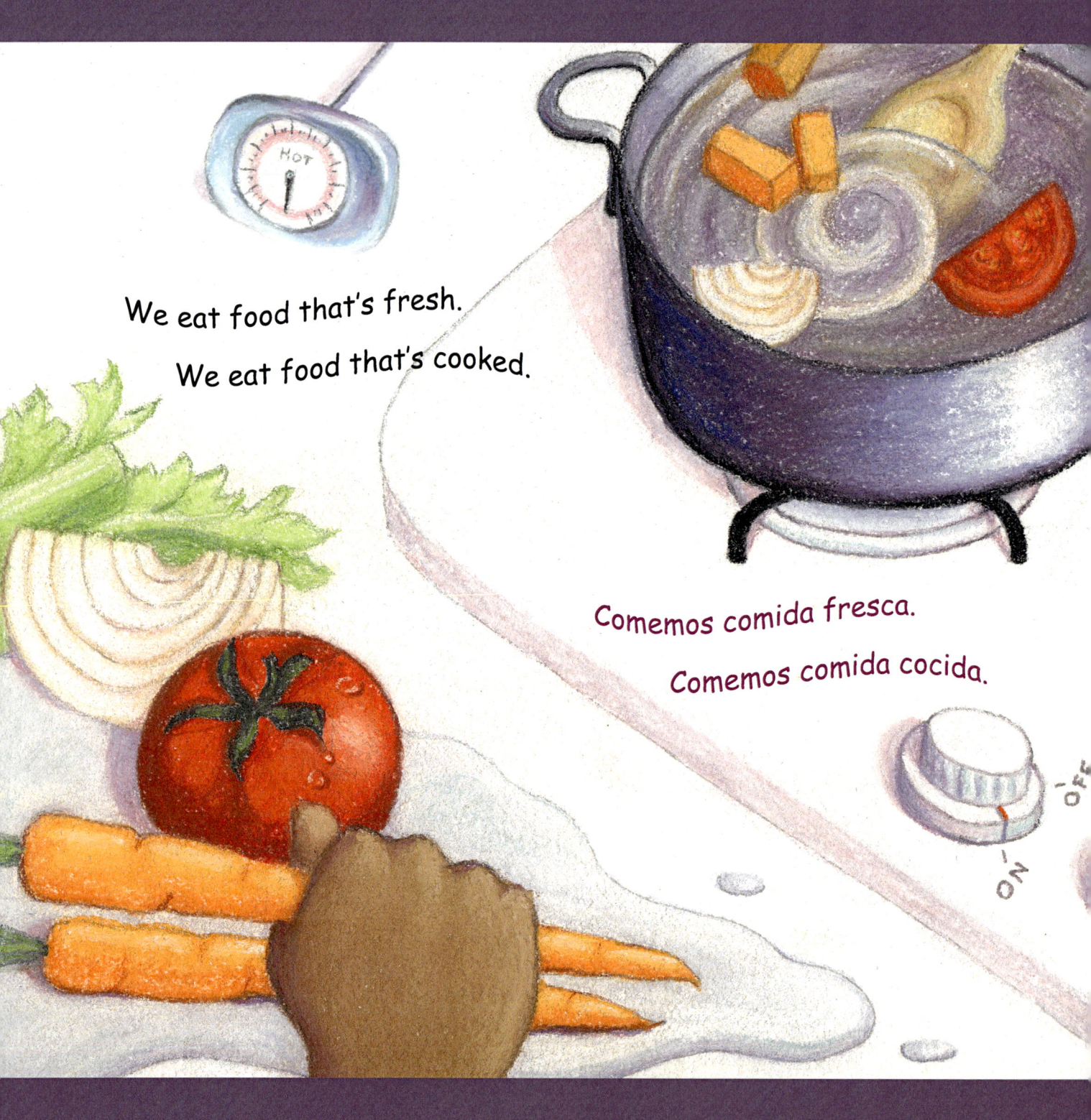

We eat food that's fresh.
We eat food that's cooked.

Comemos comida fresca.
Comemos comida cocida.

We eat food prepared from a recipe book.

Vegetable Soup

tomato celery
carrot onion
potato bay leaf

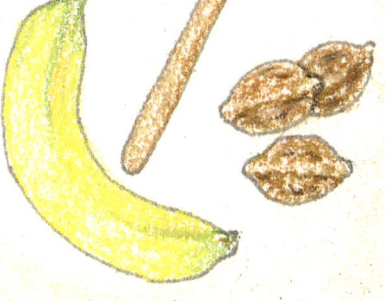

Frozen Banana

banana
wooden stick
chopped nuts

Comemos comida preparada, según un libro de cocina.

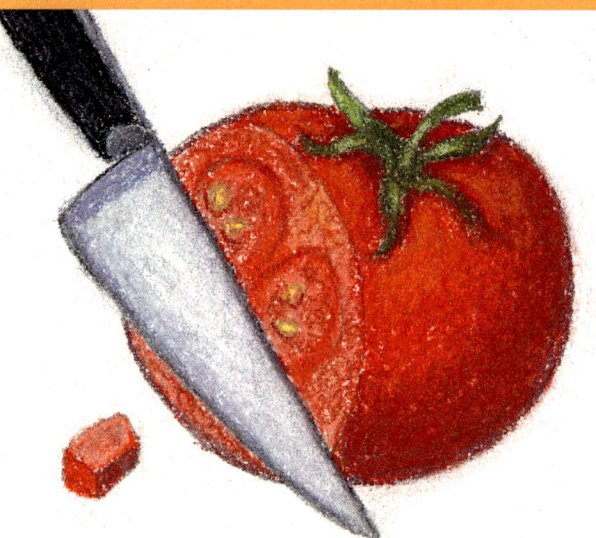
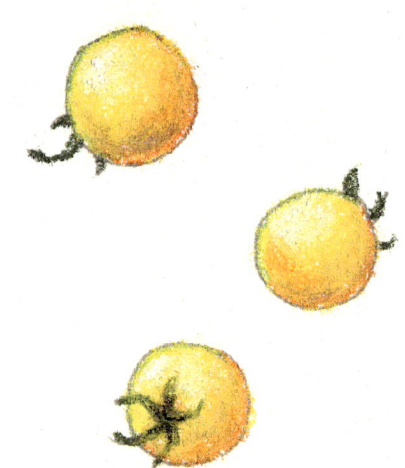

We eat food that's chopped.

We eat food that's not.

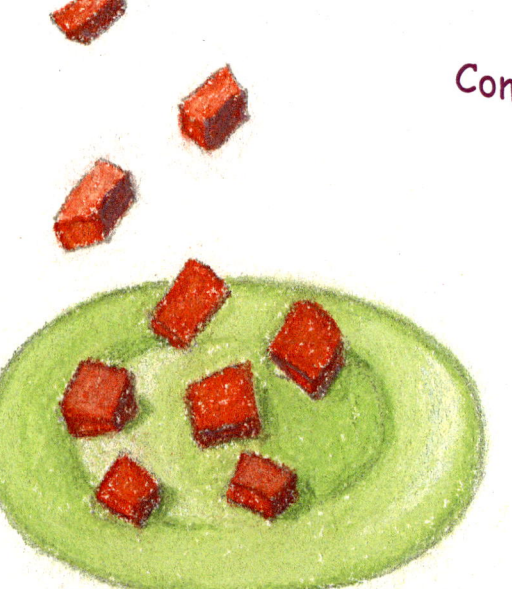

Comemos comida picada.

Comemos comida entera.

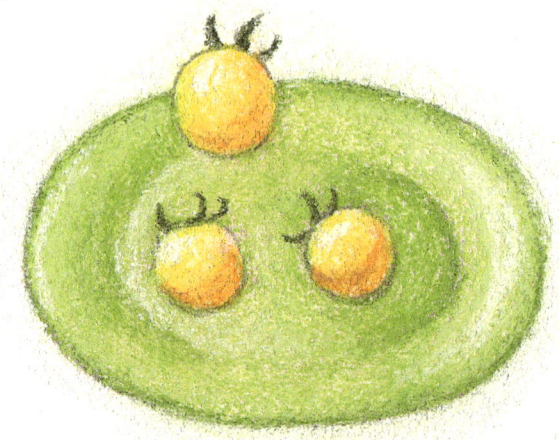

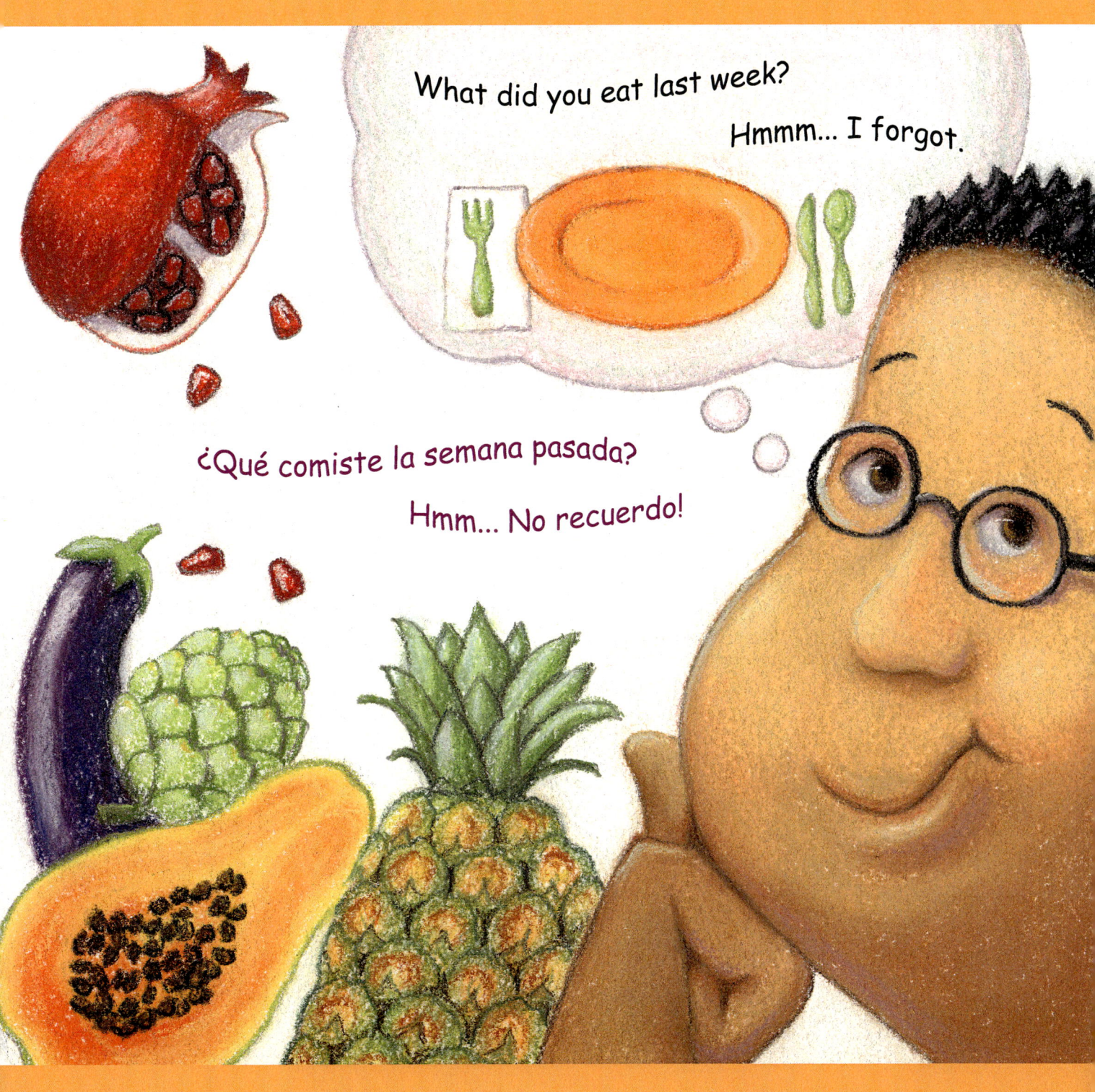

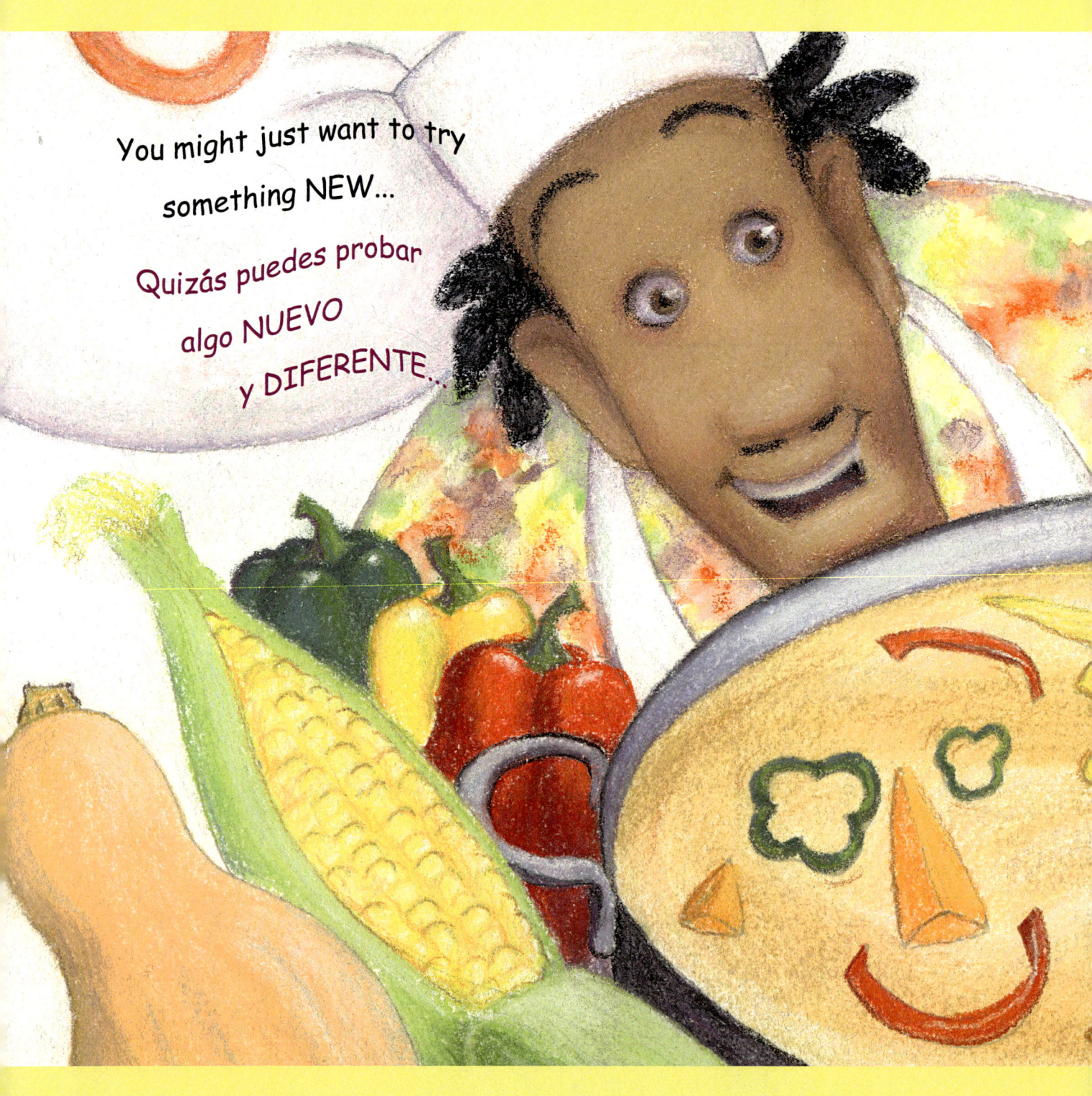

You might just want to try something NEW...

Quizás puedes probar algo NUEVO y DIFERENTE...

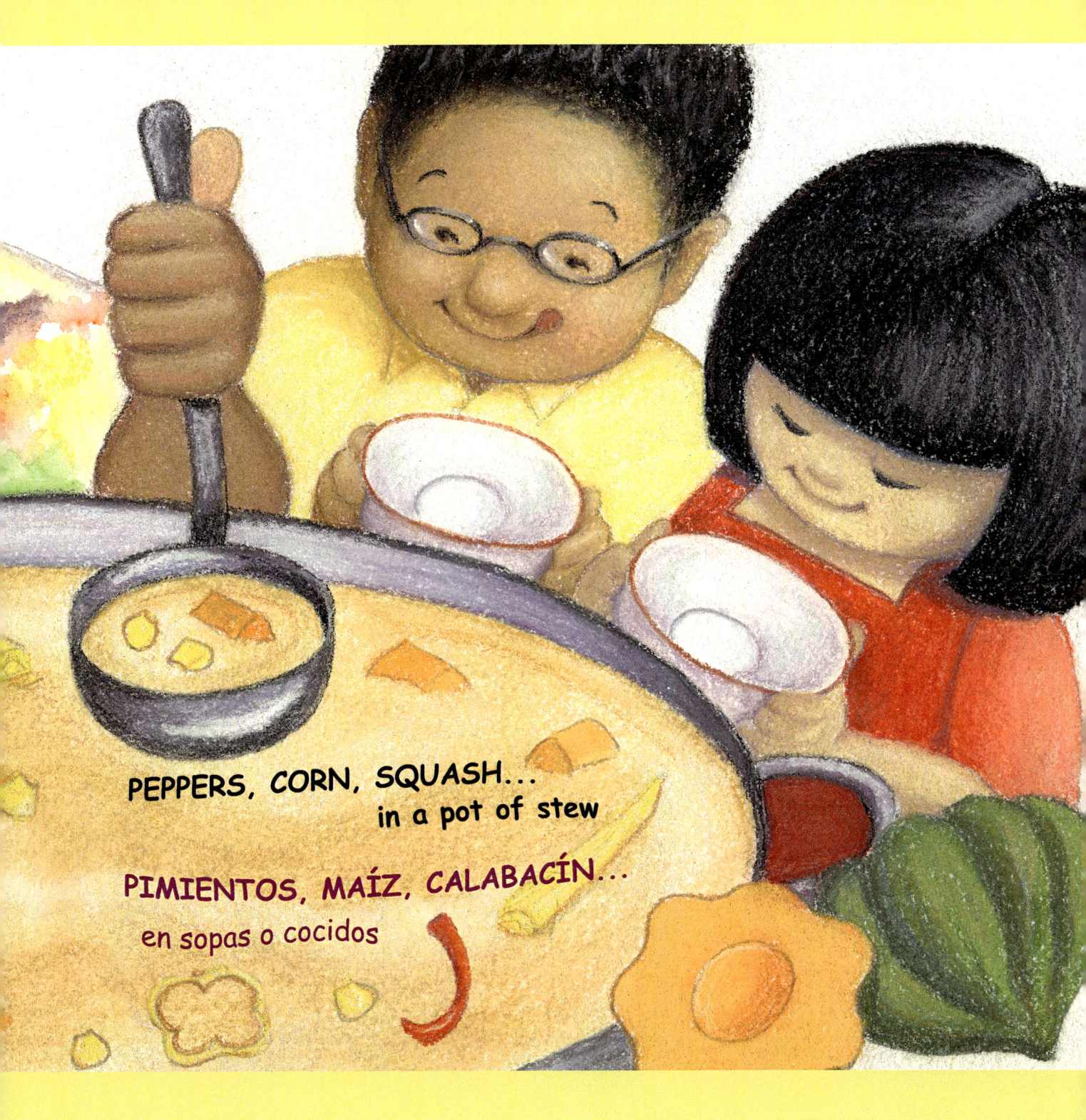

PEPPERS, CORN, SQUASH...
in a pot of stew

PIMIENTOS, MAÍZ, CALABACÍN...
en sopas o cocidos

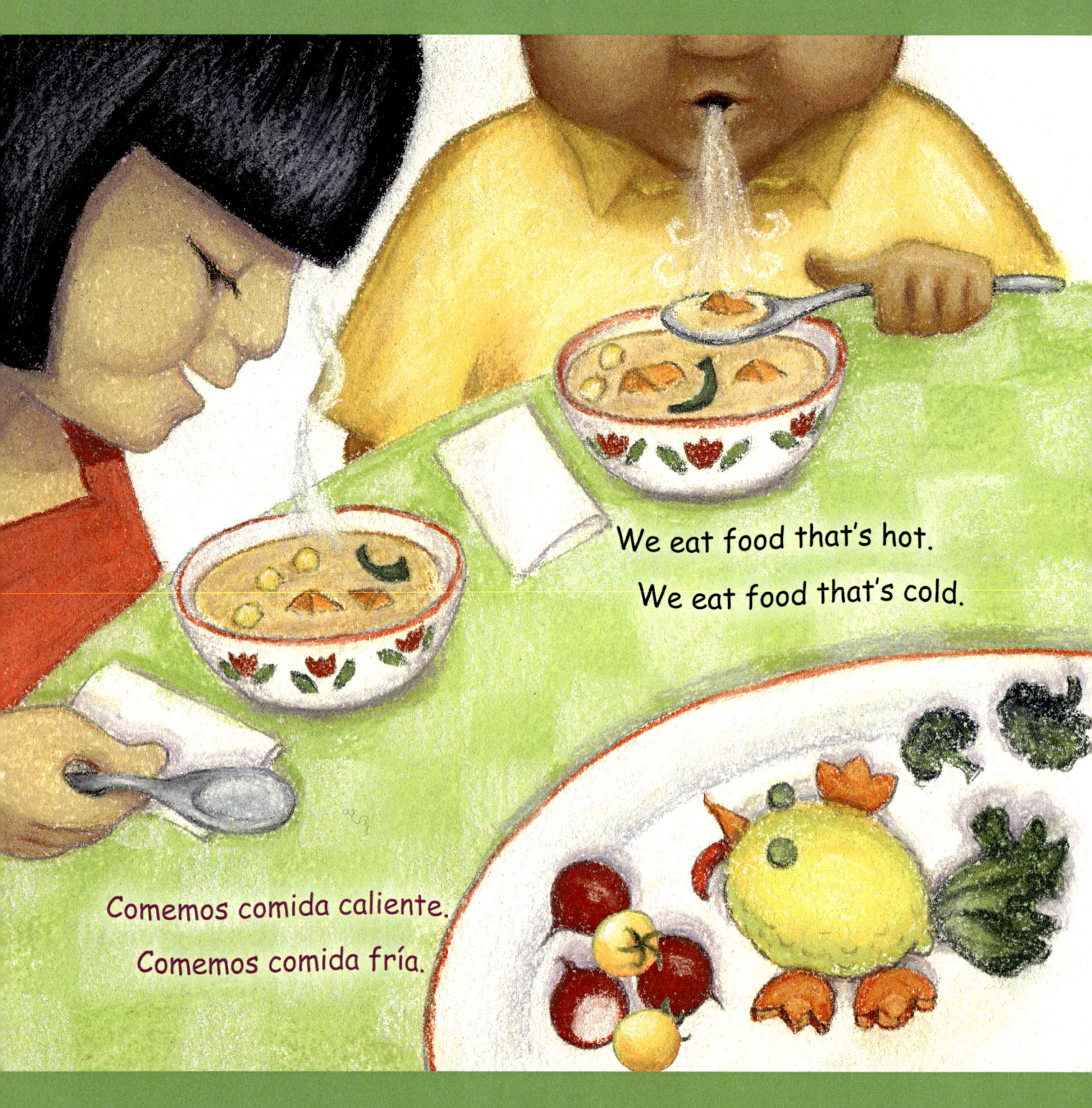

We eat food that's hot.
We eat food that's cold.

Comemos comida caliente.
Comemos comida fría.

We eat food that's grown. We eat food that's sold.

Comemos comida que cultivamos y comida que compramos.

pumpkins

cucumbers   zucchini   onions

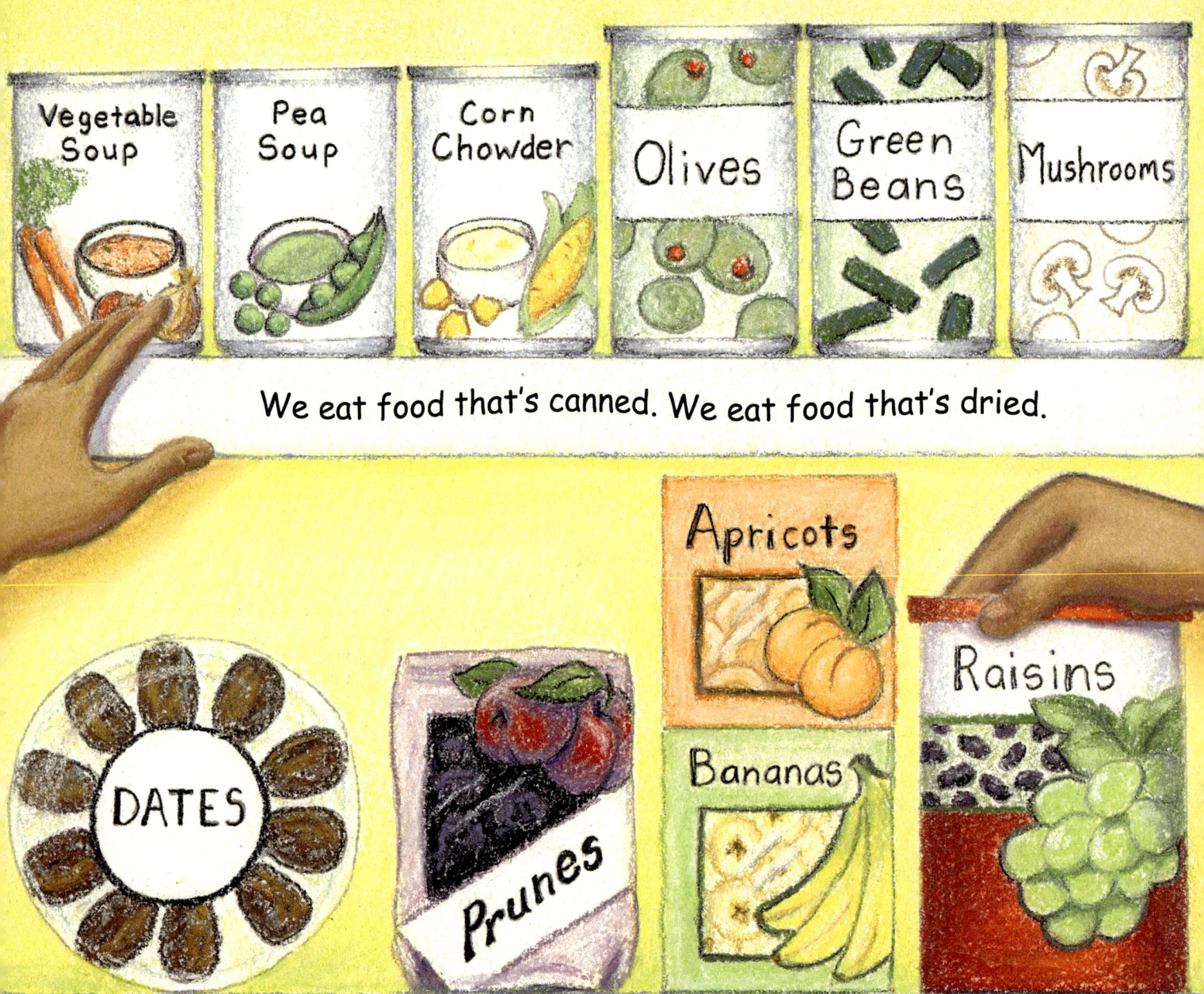

We eat food that's canned. We eat food that's dried.

Comemos comida enlatada. Comemos comida deshidratada.

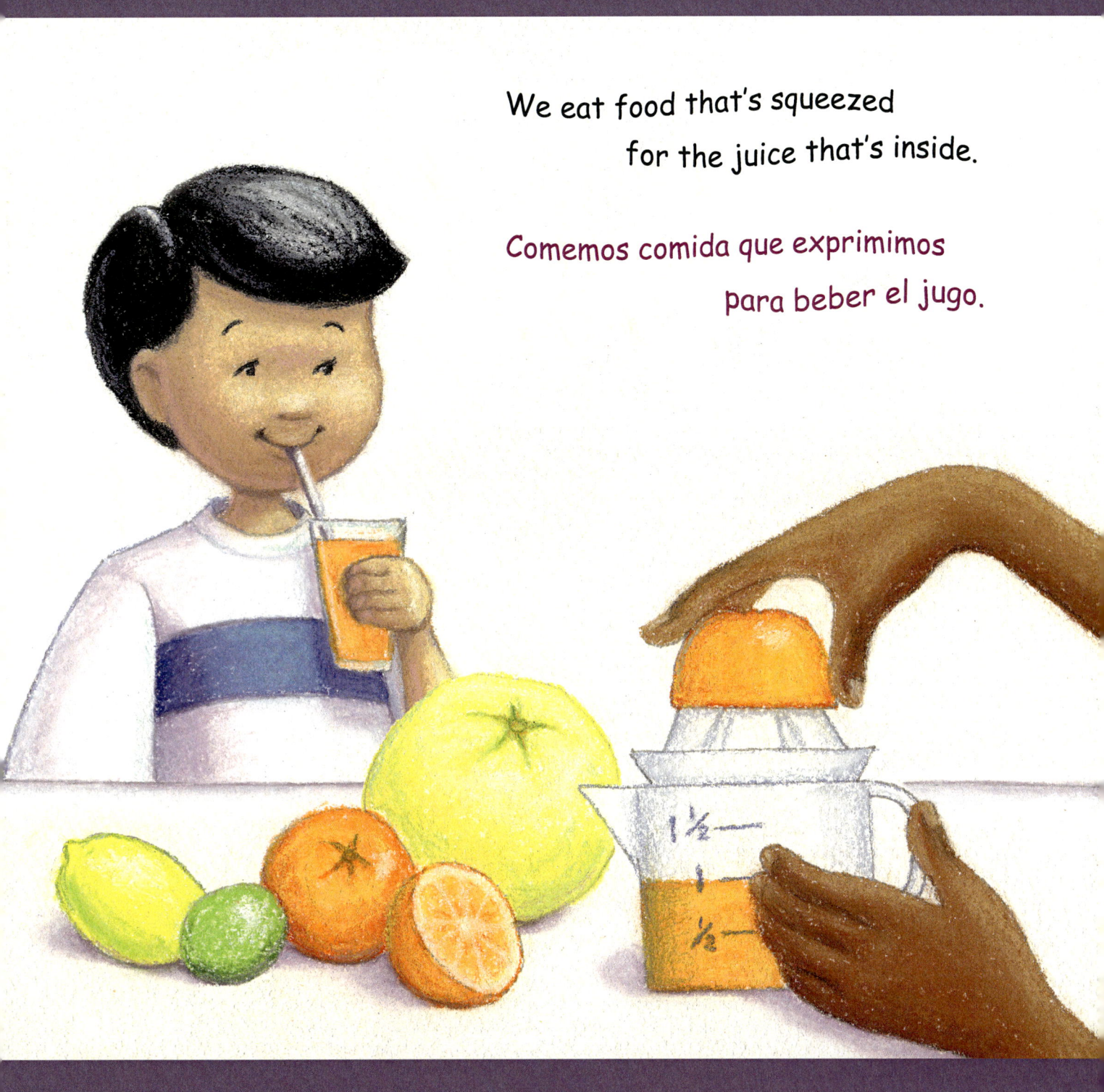

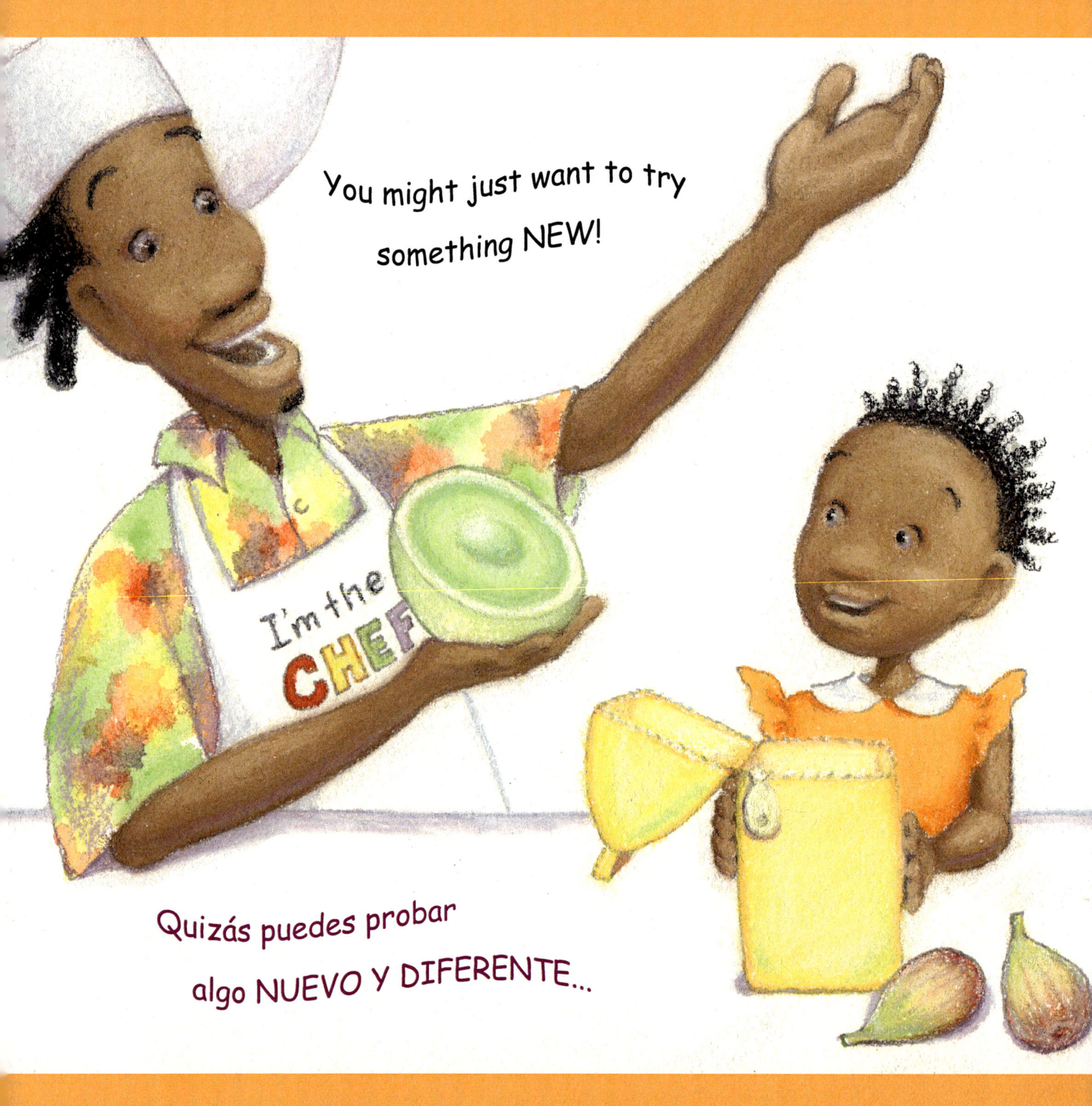

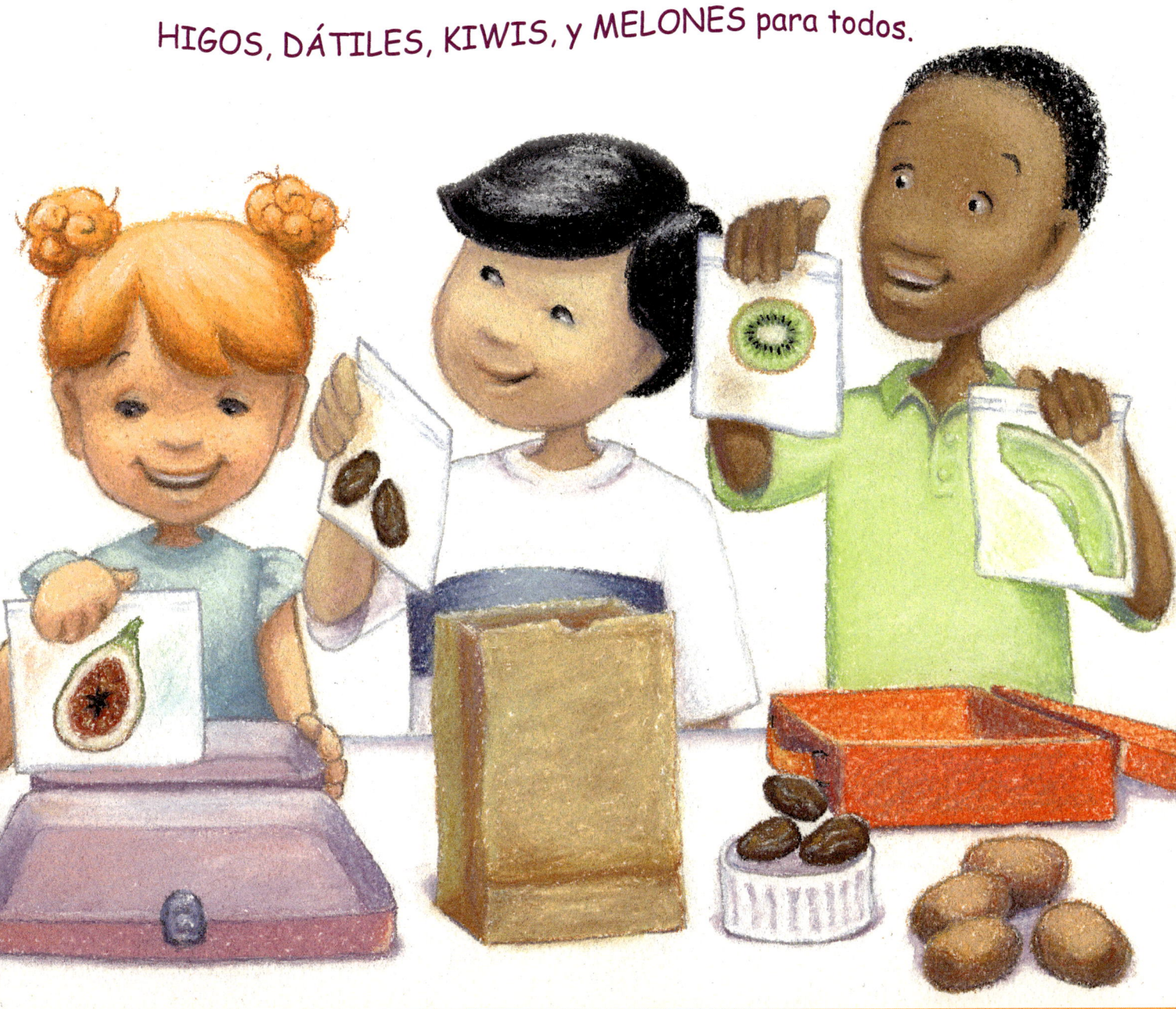

FIGS, DATES, KIWI, or some HONEYDEW.

HIGOS, DÁTILES, KIWIS, y MELONES para todos.

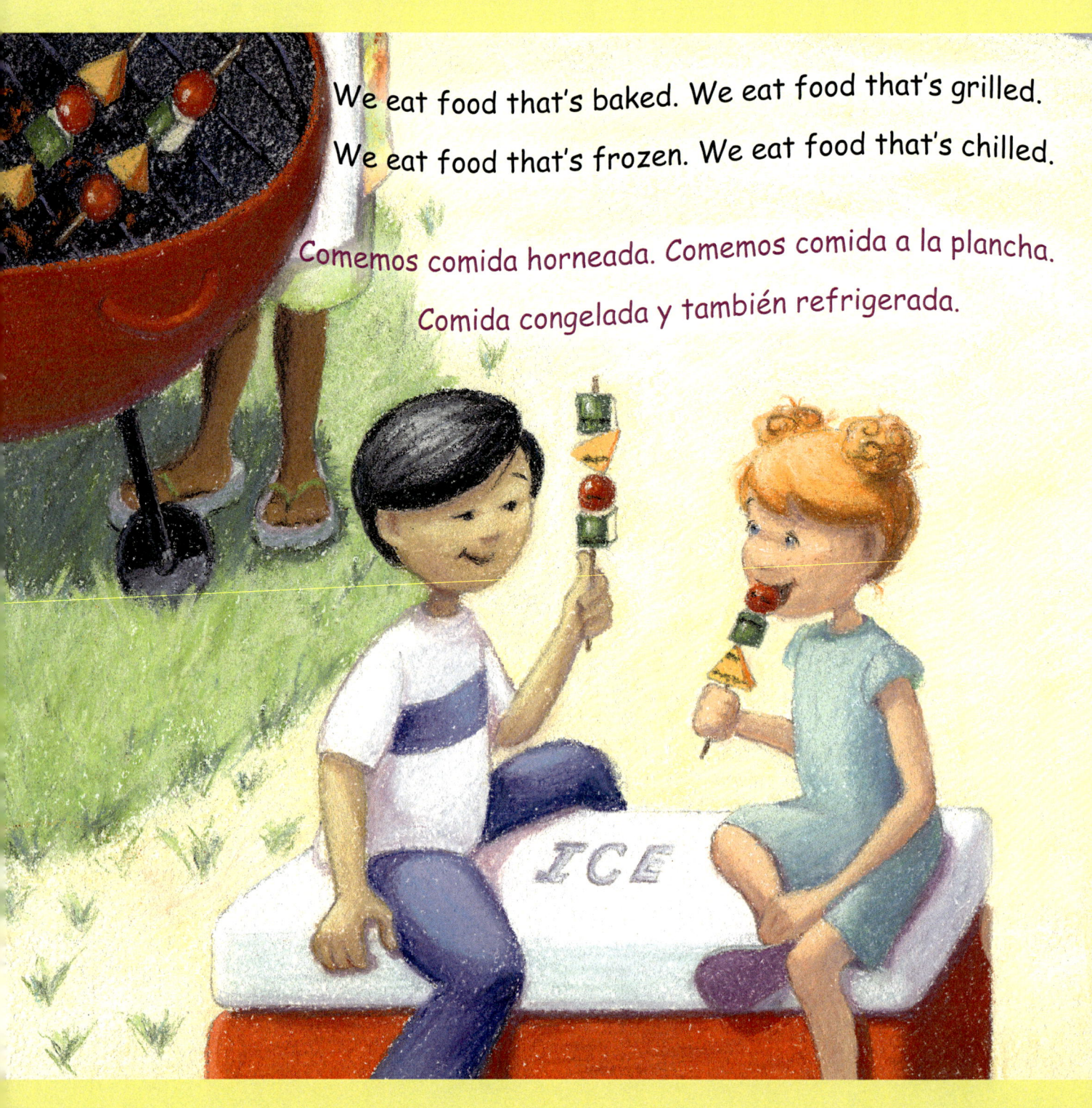

We eat food that's baked. We eat food that's grilled.
We eat food that's frozen. We eat food that's chilled.

Comemos comida horneada. Comemos comida a la plancha.
Comida congelada y también refrigerada.

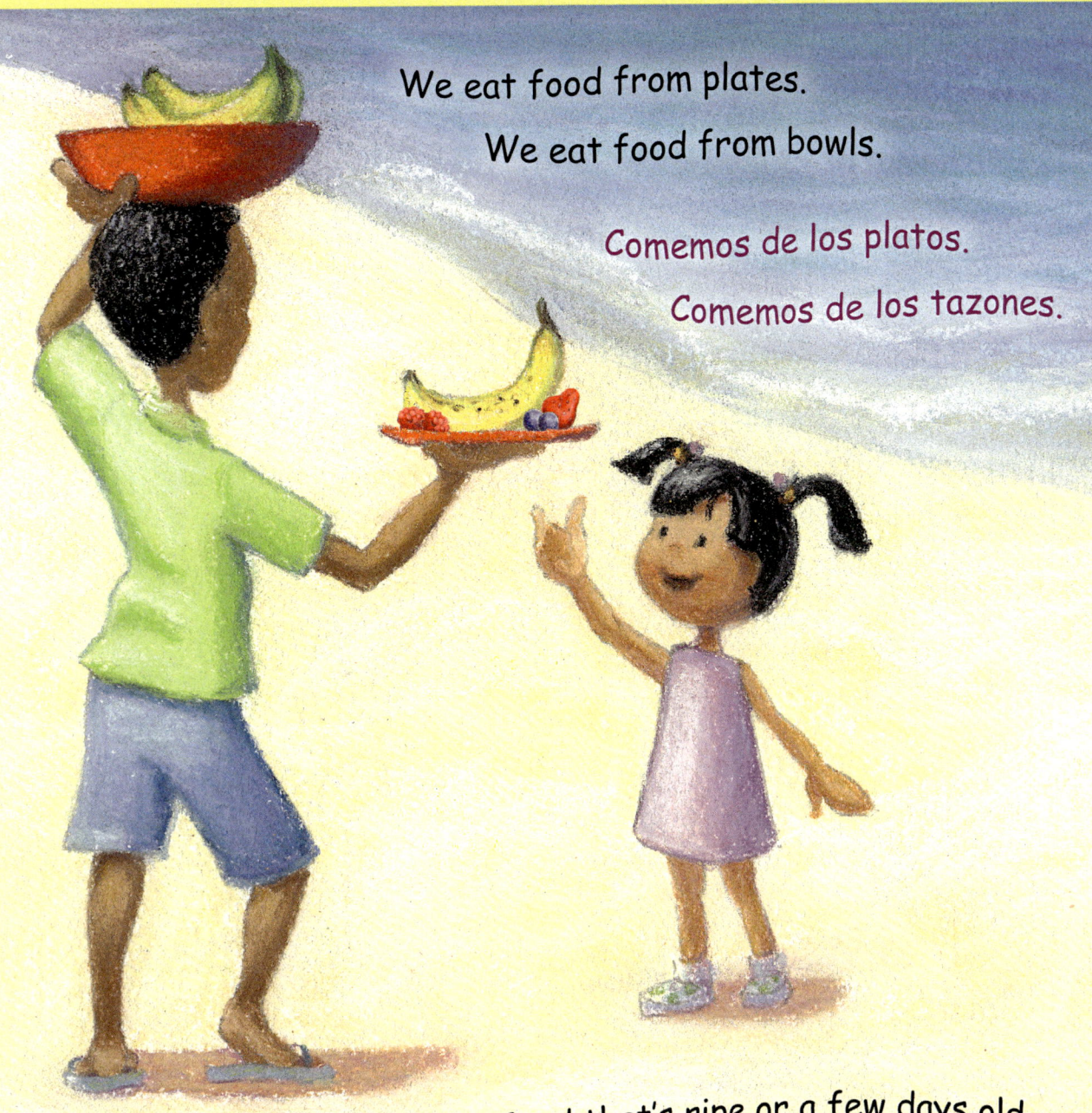

We eat food from plates.
We eat food from bowls.

Comemos de los platos.
Comemos de los tazones.

We eat food that's ripe or a few days old.
Comida que está madura o un poquito machucada.

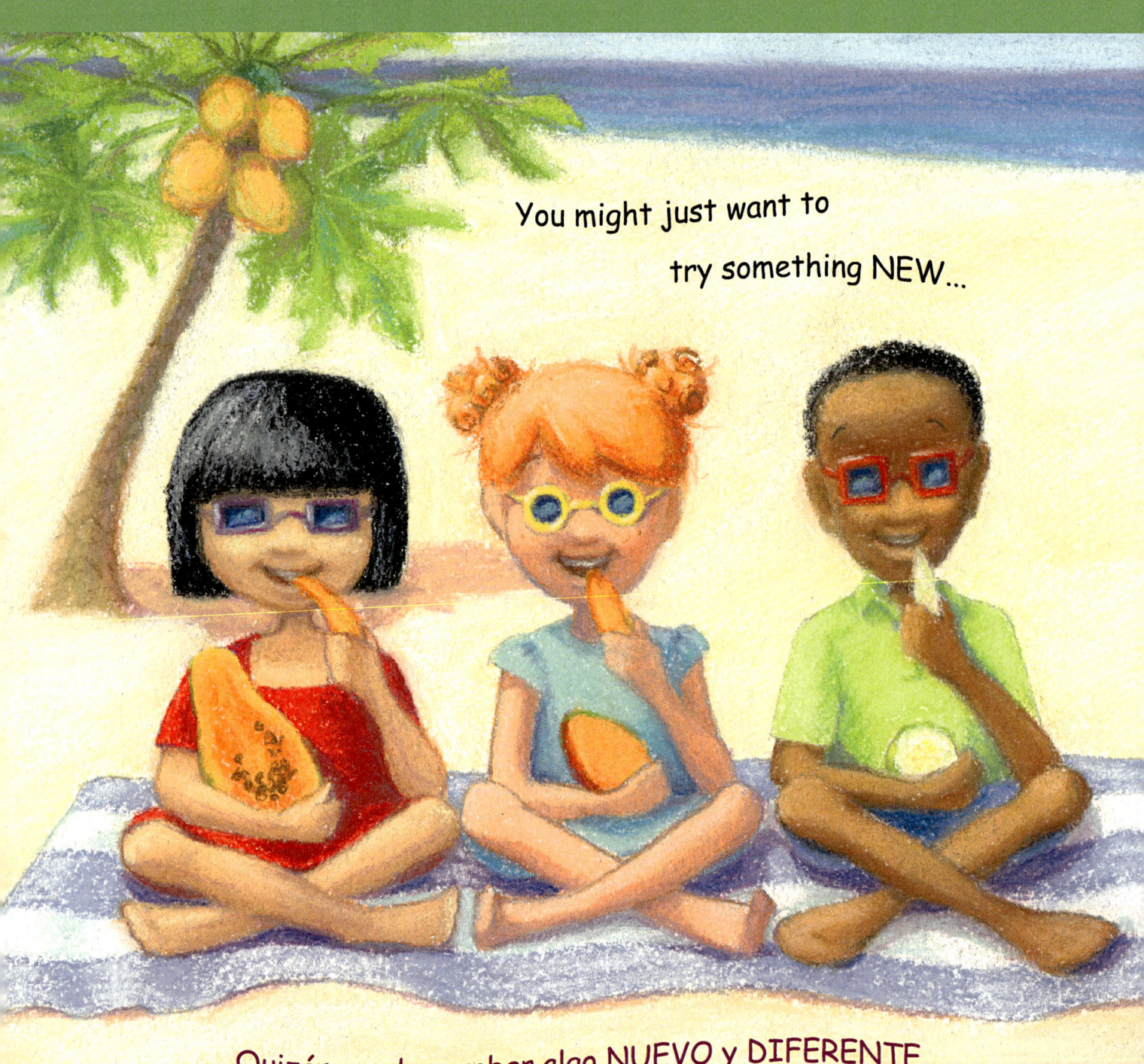

You might just want to try something NEW...

Quizás puedes probar algo NUEVO y DIFERENTE...

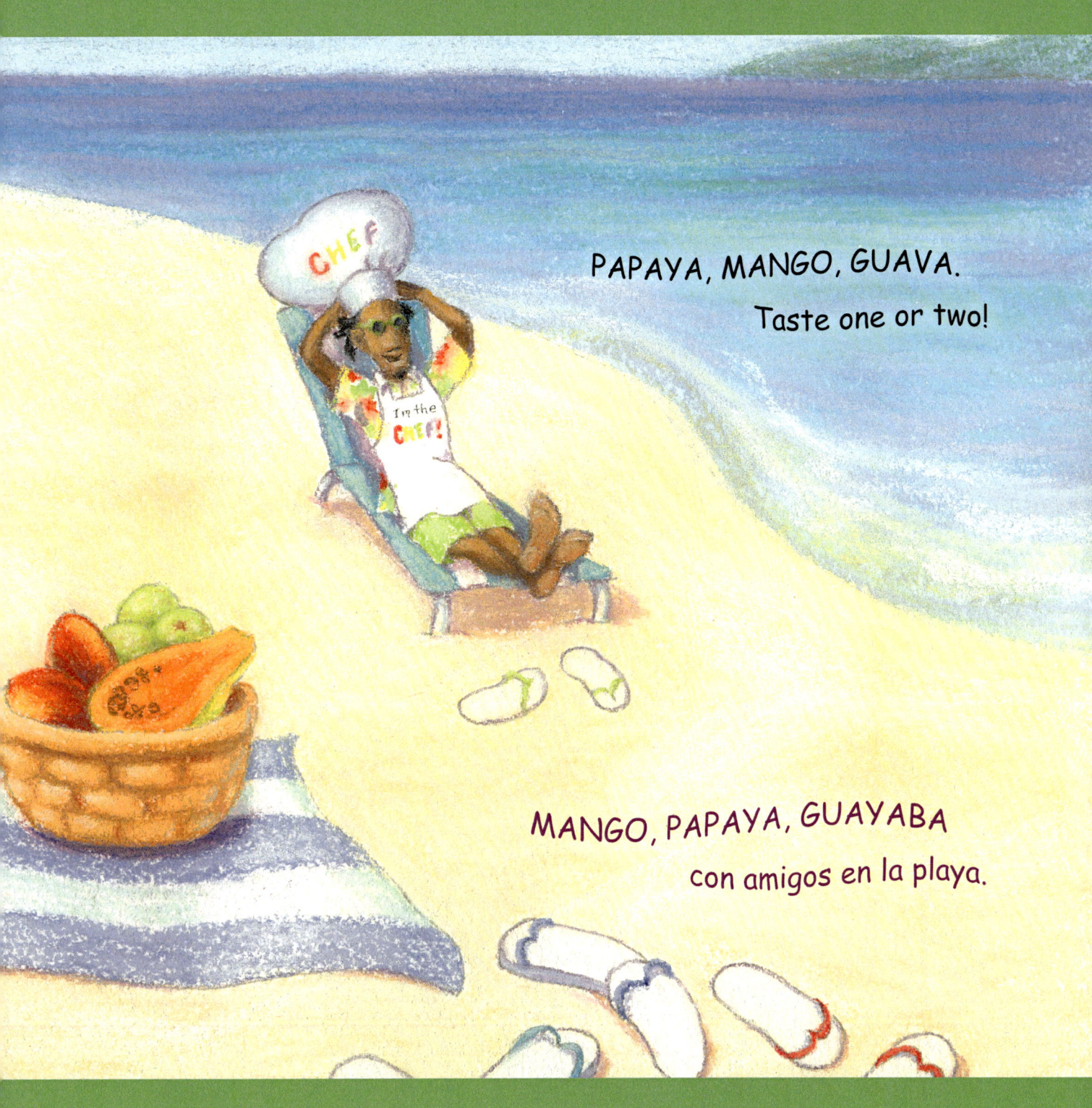

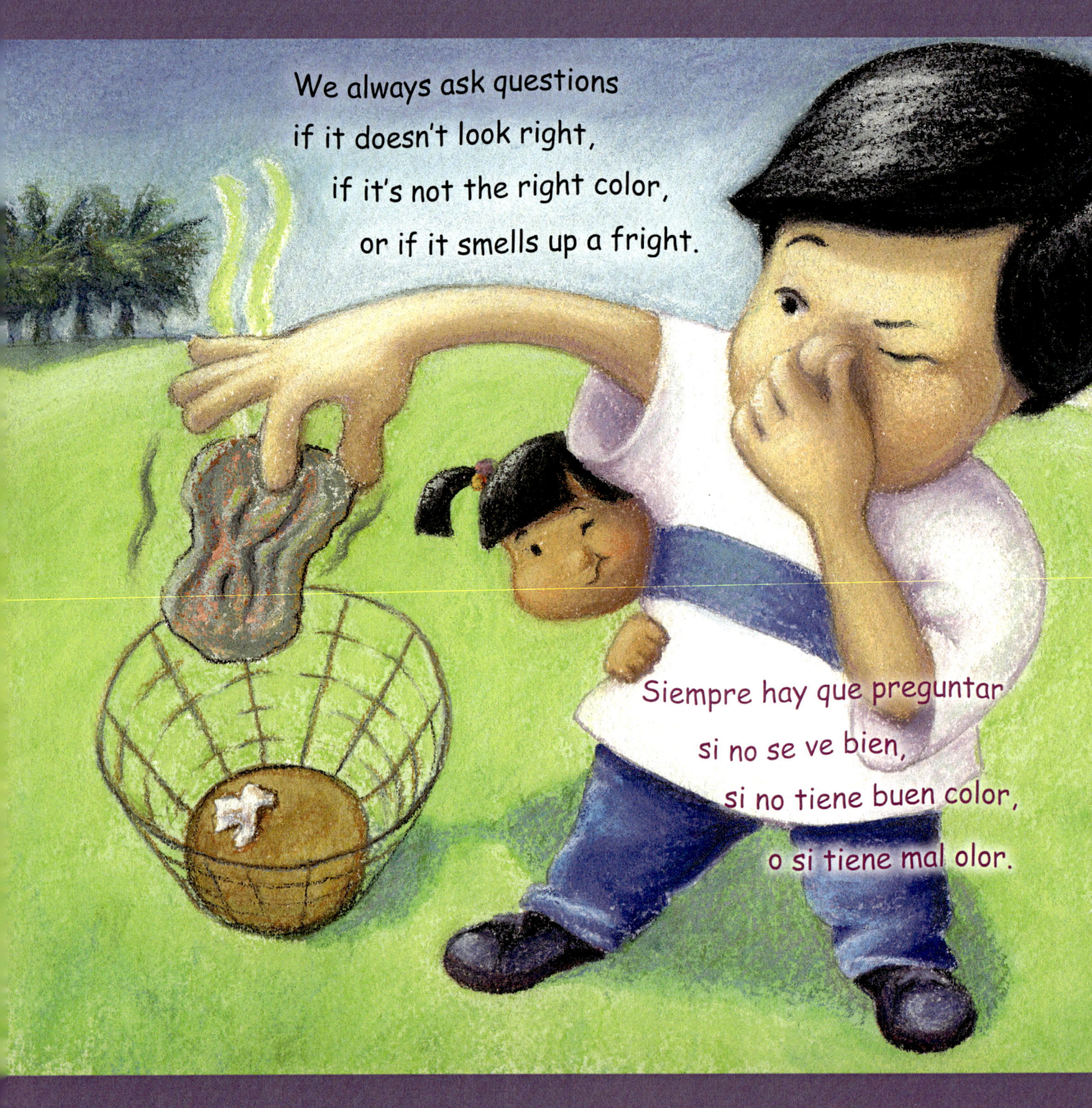

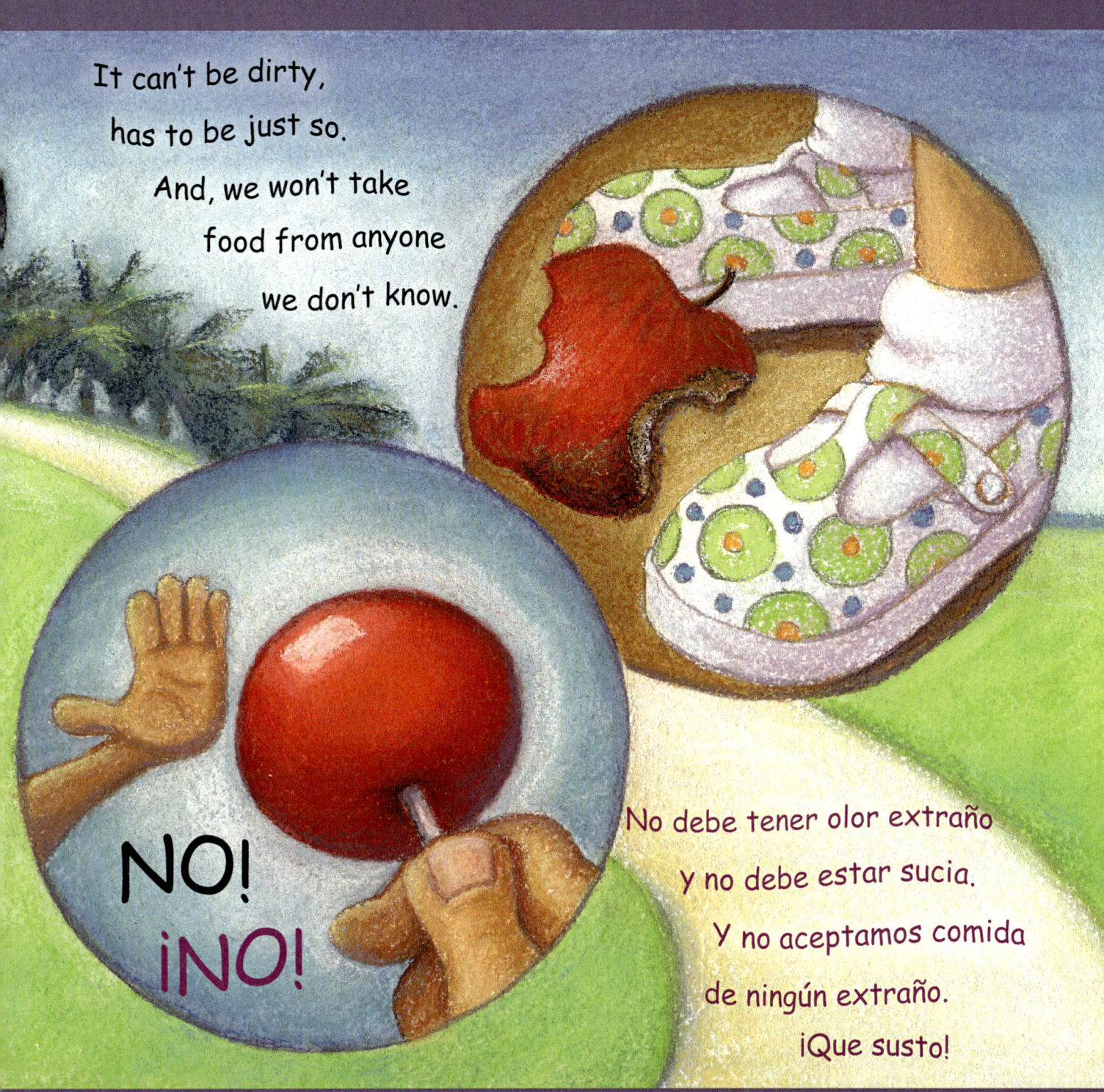

It can't be dirty,
has to be just so.
And, we won't take
food from anyone
we don't know.

NO!
¡NO!

No debe tener olor extraño
y no debe estar sucia.
Y no aceptamos comida
de ningún extraño.
¡Que susto!

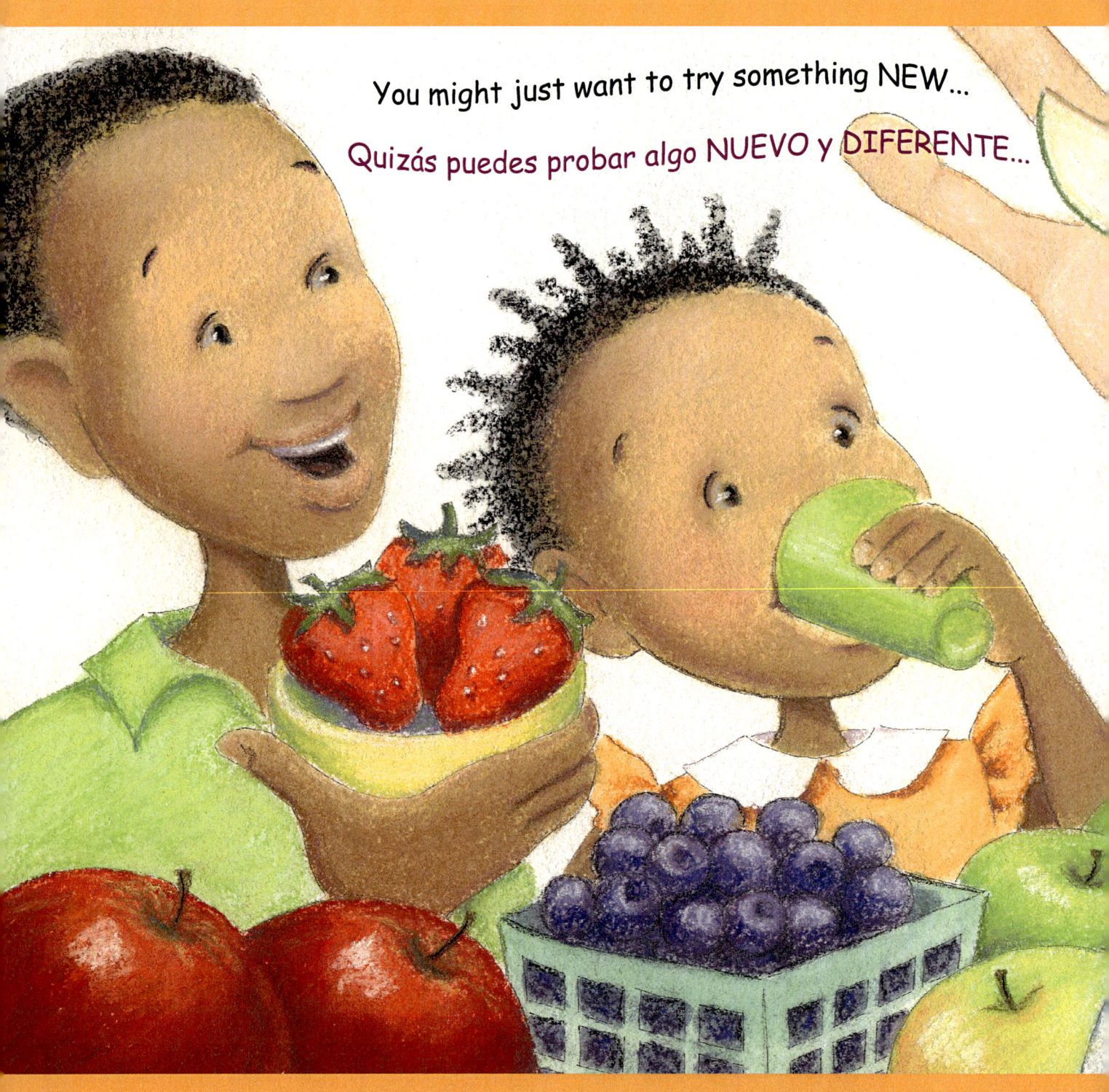

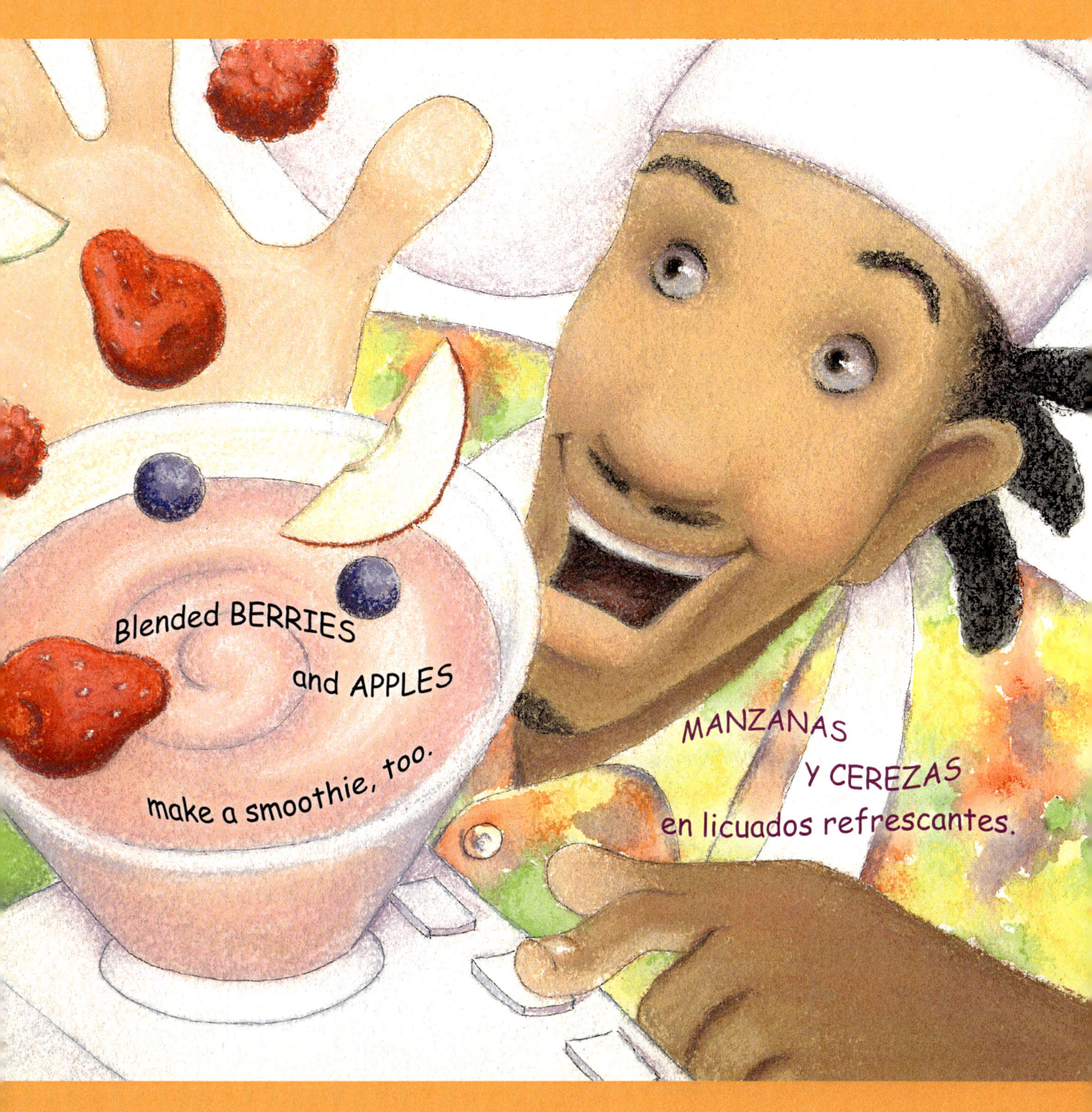

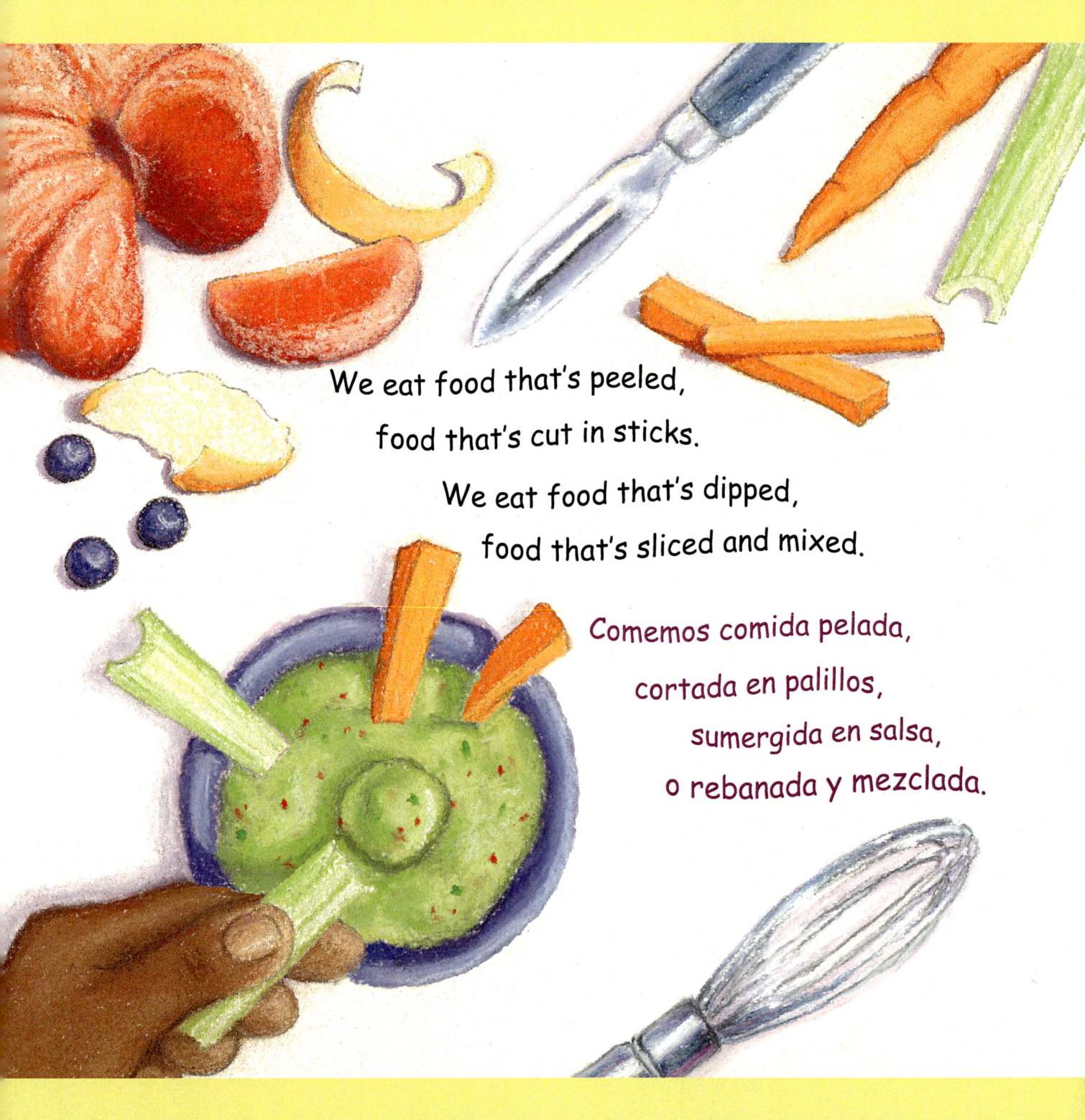

We eat food that's peeled,
food that's cut in sticks.
We eat food that's dipped,
food that's sliced and mixed.

Comemos comida pelada,
cortada en palillos,
sumergida en salsa,
o rebanada y mezclada.

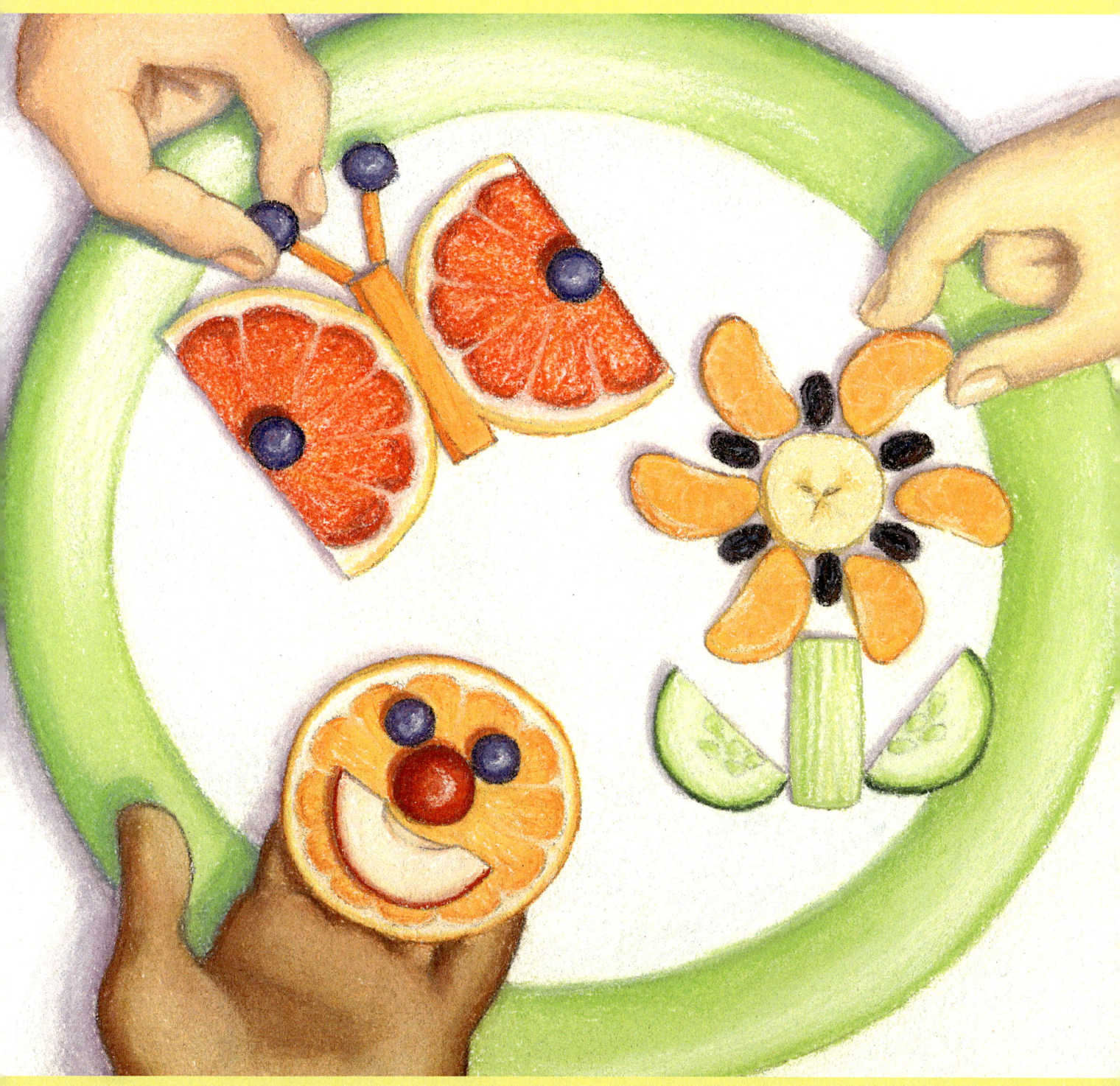

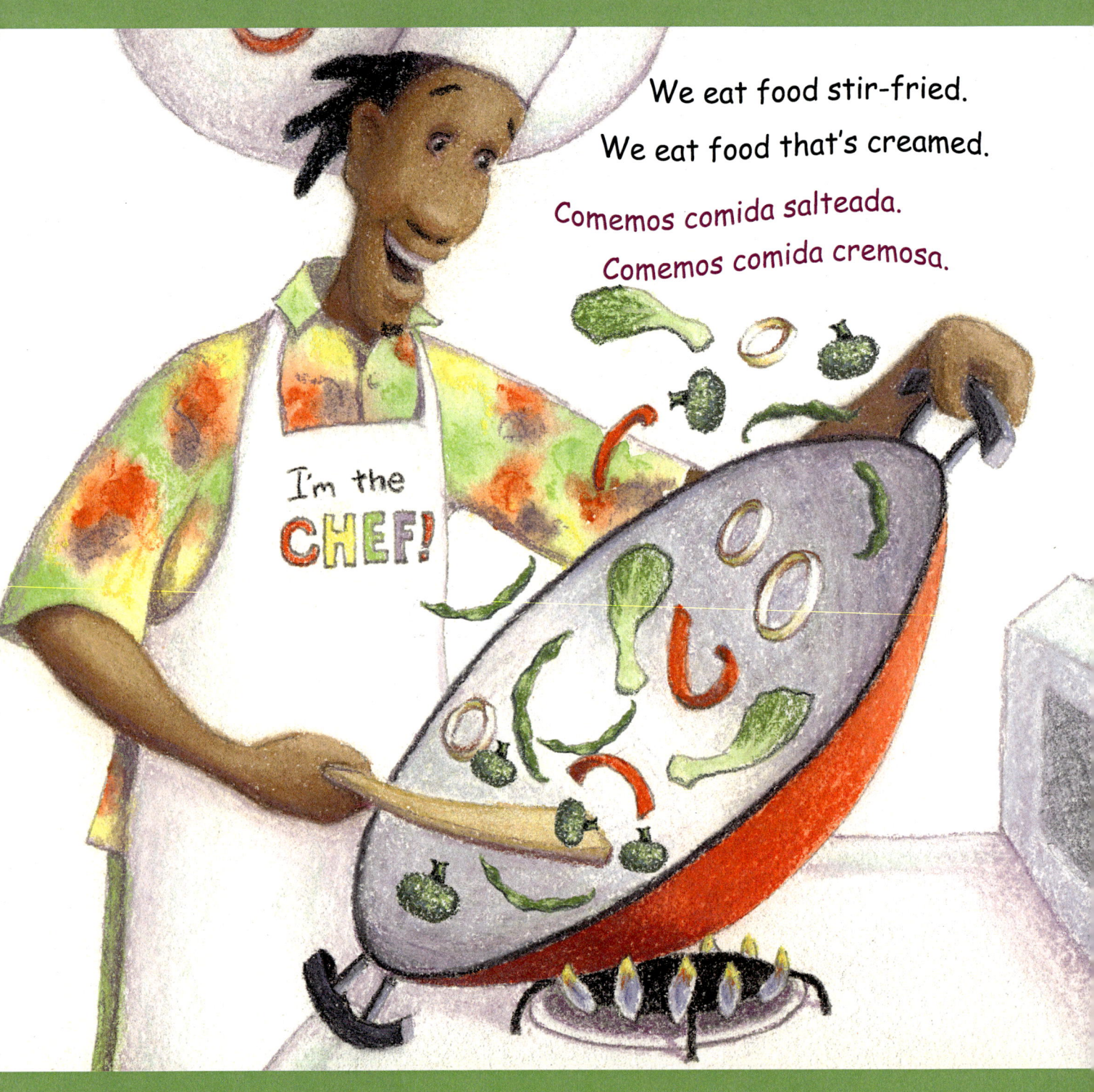

We eat food stir-fried.
We eat food that's creamed.

Comemos comida salteada.
Comemos comida cremosa.

We eat food that's boiled.
We eat food that's steamed.

Comemos comida hervida,
y al vapor cocida.

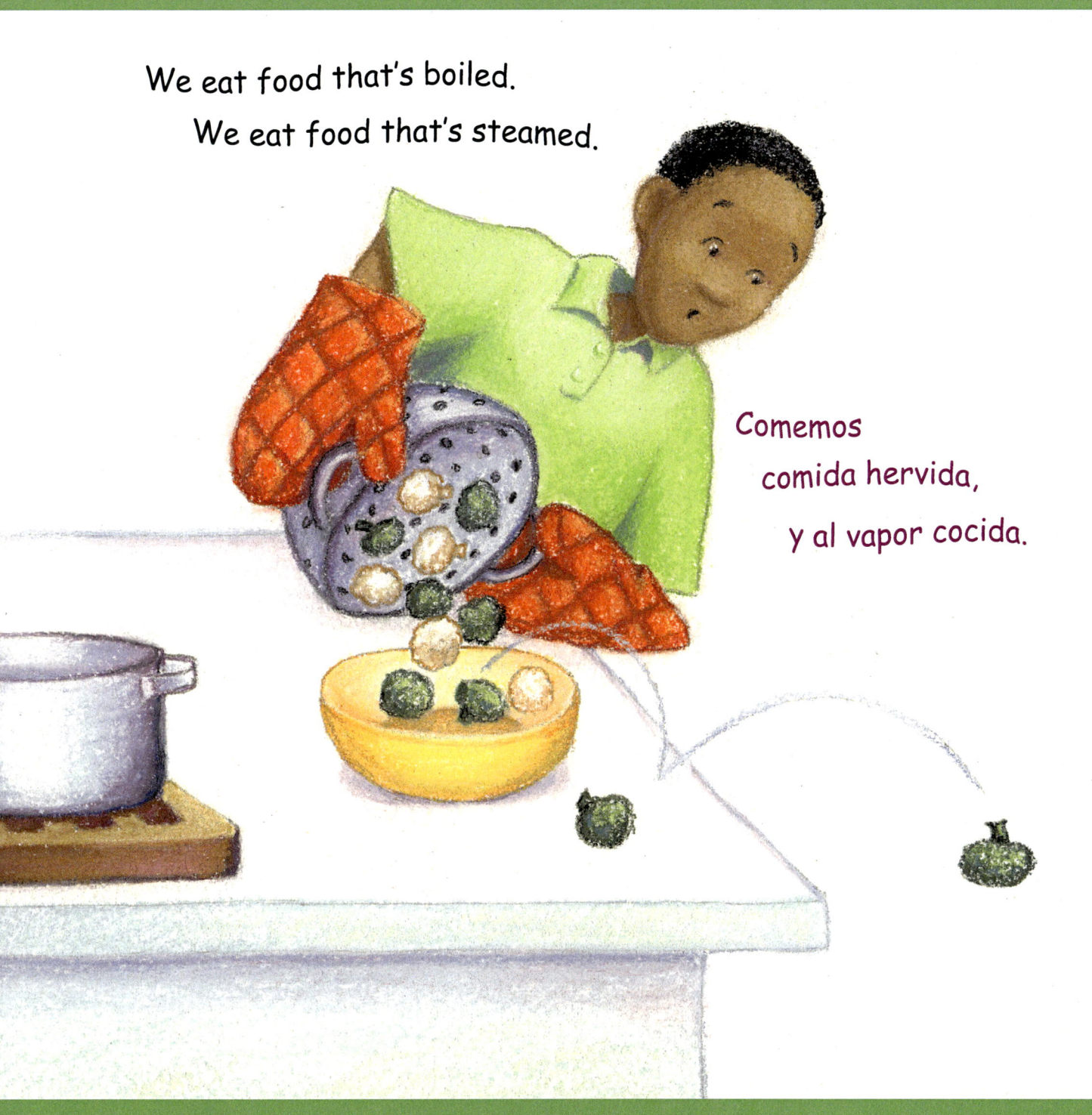

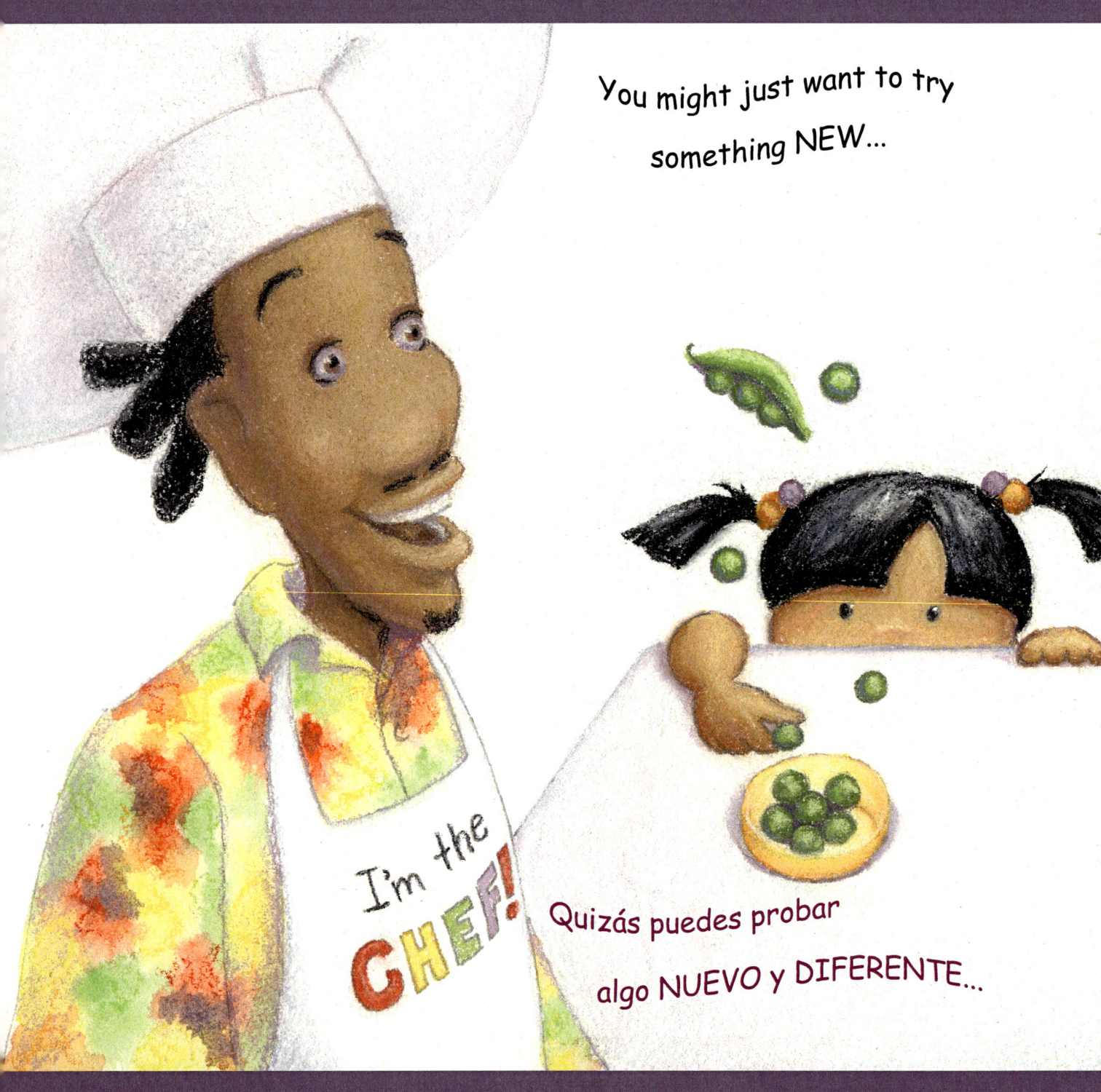

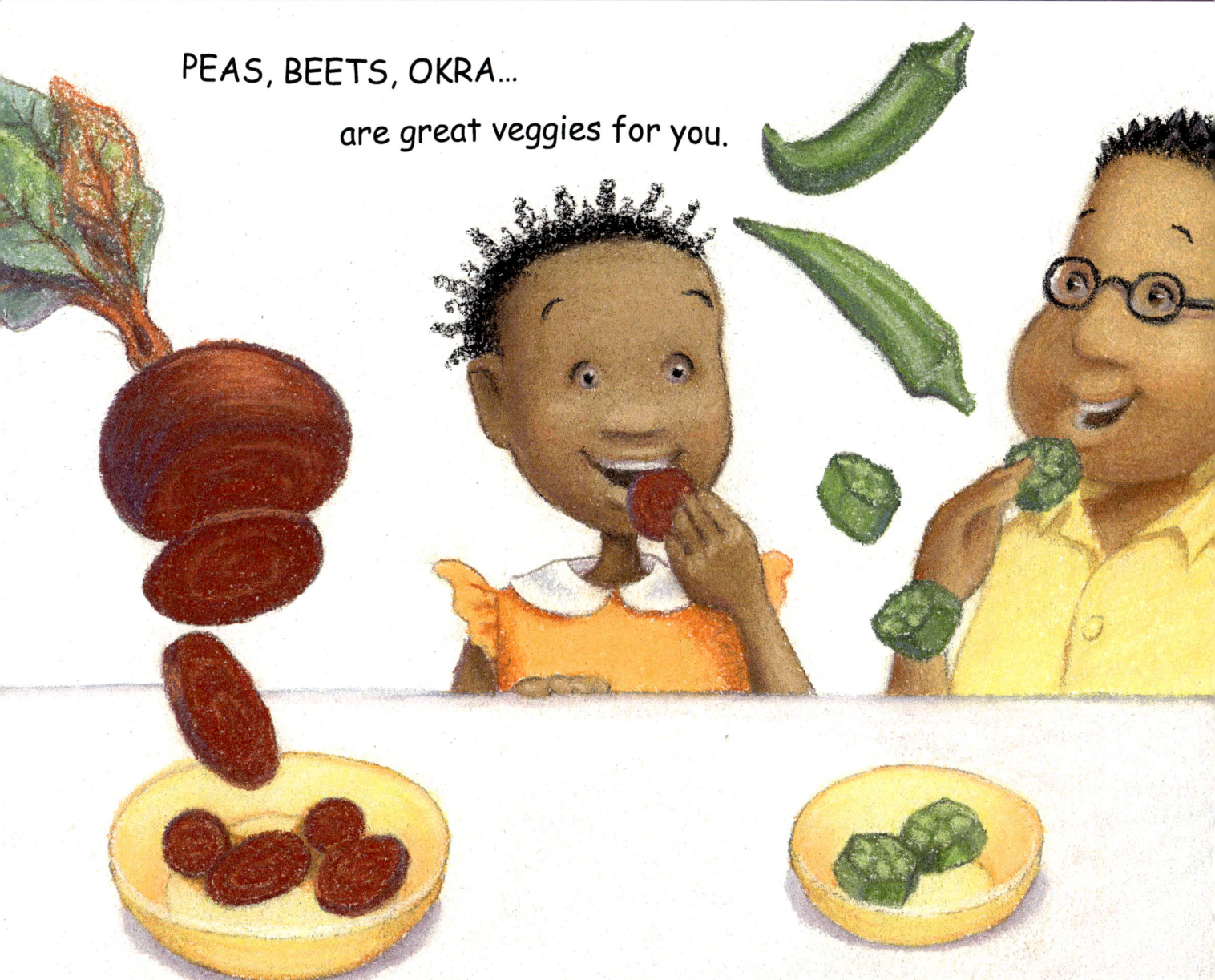

PEAS, BEETS, OKRA...
are great veggies for you.

REMOLACHA, QUINGOMBÓ, Y GUISANTES...
son buenos para todos.

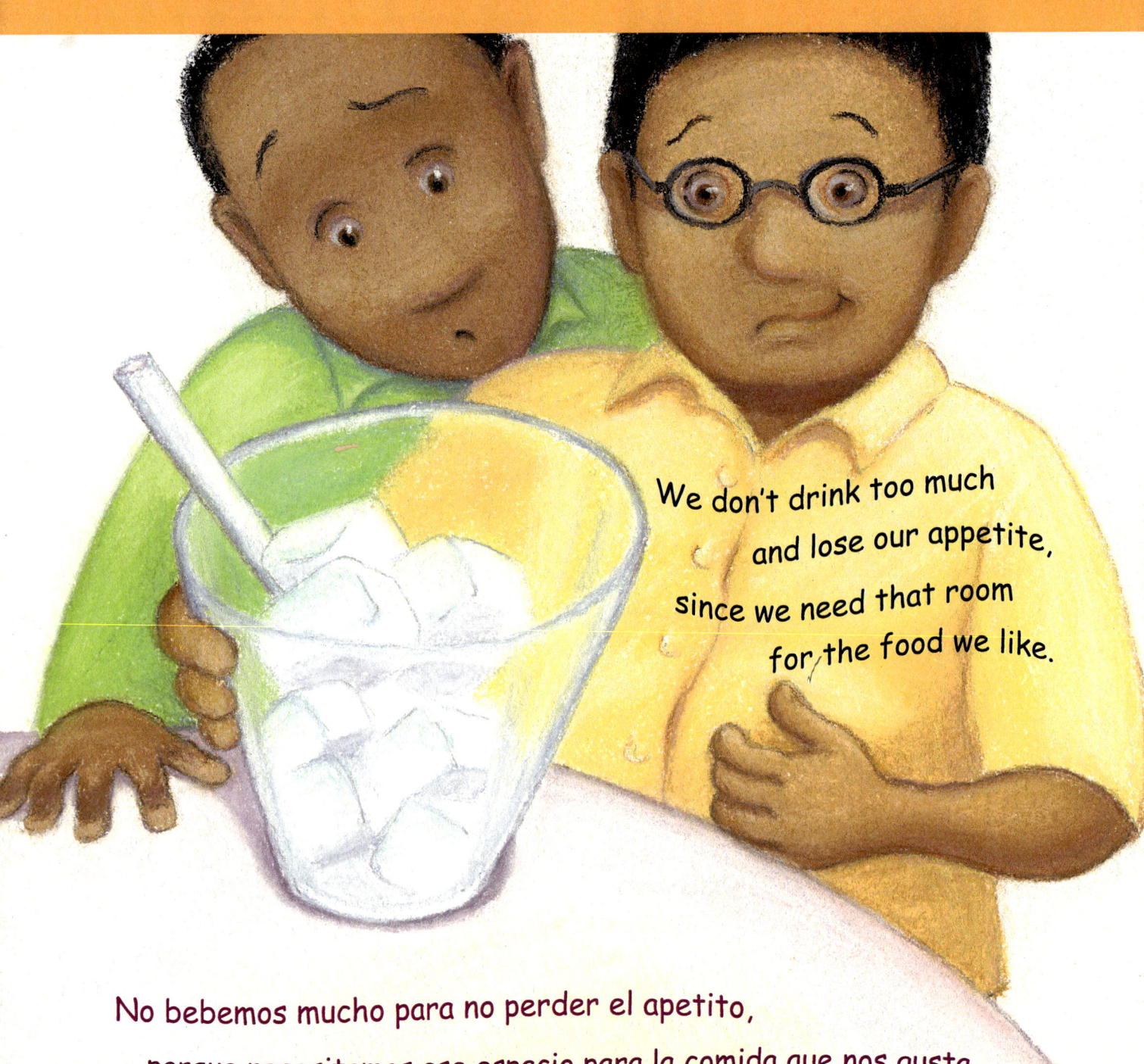

We don't drink too much and lose our appetite, since we need that room for the food we like.

No bebemos mucho para no perder el apetito, porque necesitamos ese espacio para la comida que nos gusta.

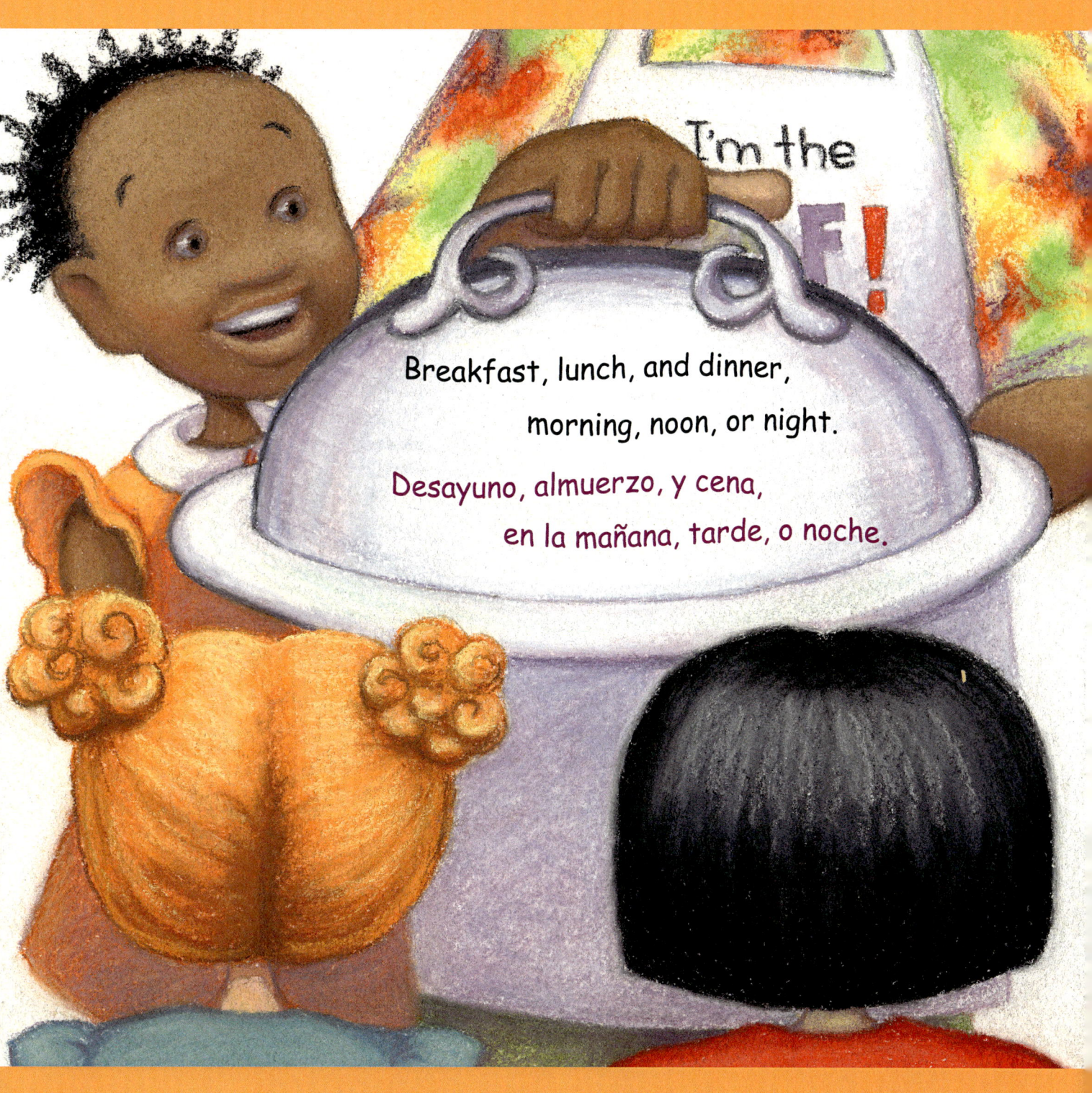

Breakfast, lunch, and dinner,
morning, noon, or night.

Desayuno, almuerzo, y cena,
en la mañana, tarde, o noche.

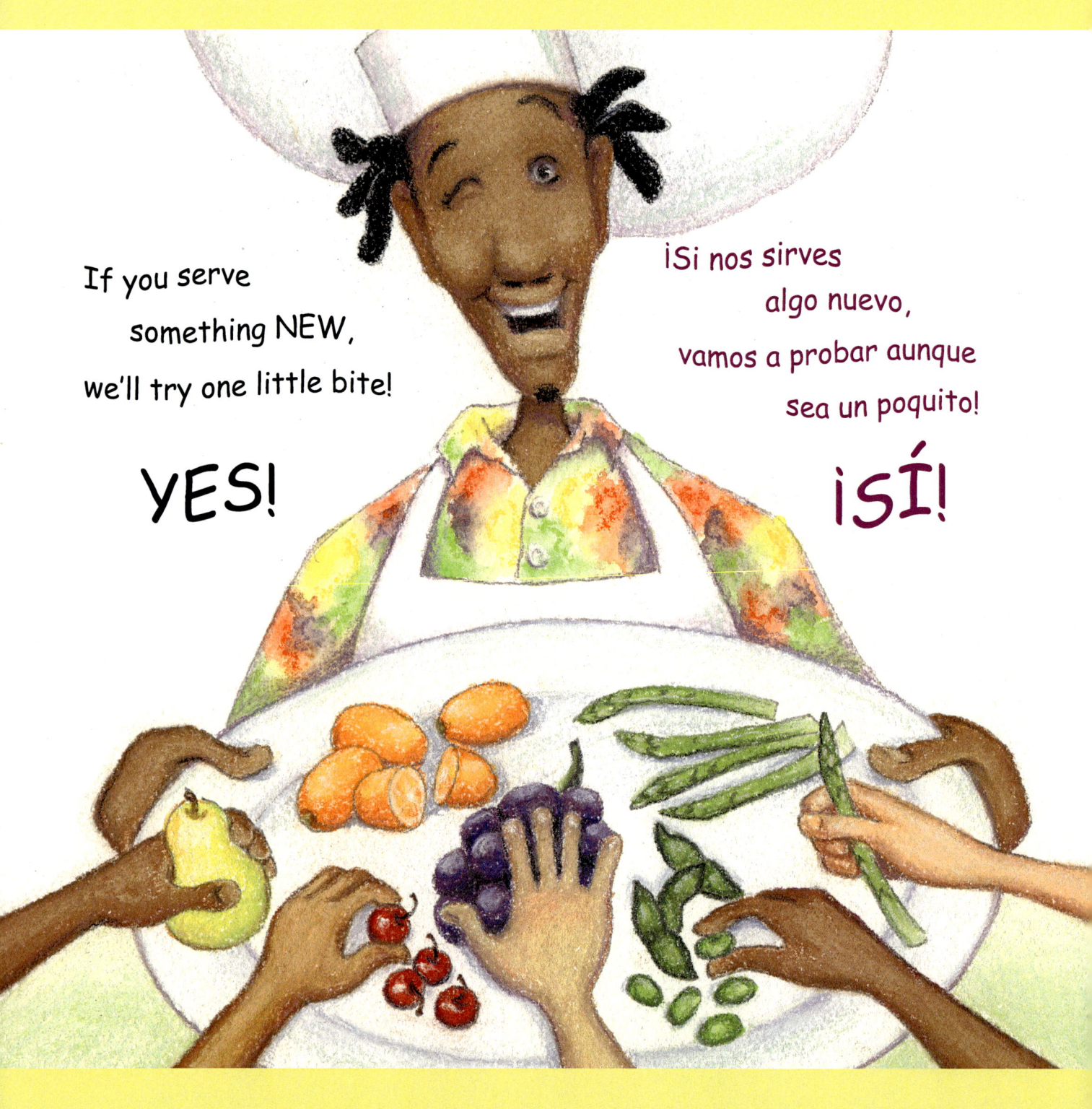

Made in the USA
San Bernardino, CA
18 July 2017